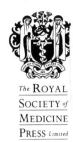

The ROYAL
SOCIETY of
MEDICINE
PRESS Limited

Parkinson's Disease

in Practice

Carl E Clarke

Reader in Clinical Neurology and Consultant
Neurologist at City Hospital NHS Trust and
University of Birmingham, UK

British Library Cataloguing in Publication Data
A catalogue record for this book is available from the British Library

ISBN 1-85315-486-5
ISSN 1473-6845

Typeset by Phoenix Photosetting, Chatham, Kent
Printed in Great Britain by Latimer Trend & Company Ltd, Plymouth

Dedication

To my wife, Jan, and daughter, Helen, for their love and support
without which this book would never have been written

About the author

Dr Carl E Clarke is a Reader in Clinical Neurology and Consultant Neurologist at City Hospital NHS Trust and the University of Birmingham, UK. He studied Anatomy and Medicine at the University of Manchester and completed his postgraduate training in Manchester and Yorkshire.

He has been involved in Parkinson's disease research for 14 years. His current interests include systematic reviews of clinical trials in Parkinson's disease and large-scale pragmatic clinical trials such as PDMED and PDSURG.

Preface

The pace of change in the pharmacology and surgery for Parkinson's disease has been phenomenal over the past 10 years. New types and classes of drug have been introduced, and in some cases discontinued, and surgical techniques have undergone a considerable revival. How can the busy generalist, medical or paramedical keep up with such developments?

This book reviews the entire spectrum of Parkinson's disease in a concise format, with particular emphasis on current therapeutics. It will be especially useful to the general practitioner with only four or five patients with Parkinson's disease but who needs to 'dip in' to or browse through a short reference book on the condition. It should also prove valuable to undergraduate and postgraduate students of medicine, pharmacology and pharmacy. In addition, the burgeoning numbers of Parkinson's disease nurse specialists in the UK should find the book of value, both during their training and in the field thereafter. Paramedical therapists from all of the specialties treating Parkinson's disease should also find this a useful source of reference.

In line with the current enthusiasm for evidence-based practice, each chapter reviews the current evidence in the area in question. I have highlighted key points and facts, and have tried to provide practical advice and useful further reading lists. Many of the recommendations from the therapy chapters are brought together in the final chapter on formal management guidelines.

Grateful thanks are due to Mrs R Mitchell, Dr H Benamer, Britannia Pharmaceuticals and Medtronic for providing illustrations. I would also like to thank Peter Altman and the staff at the Royal Society of Medicine Press for their help.

Carl E Clarke
August 2001

Contents

1. Epidemiology

Incidence and prevalence
Mortality

Incidence and prevalence

Incidence is the measure of the number of new cases of a disease occurring over a set period of time for a given location. Incidence rates are not affected by disease survival but are subject to bias according to methods of ascertainment and case definition. The latter point is particularly apposite in idiopathic Parkinson's disease (PD) because of the difficulties in differential diagnosis (discussed below). Only 10 such studies have been performed in PD with crude incidence rates ranging between 4.5 and 21/100,000 population/annum. Interestingly, in the stable population of Rochester, Minnesota, US, the incidence of PD varied little between 1945 and 1979 with a range of 16 to 21/100,000/annum.

> Incidence = number of new cases/year. Incidence of PD is 18/100,000 population; about 10,000 new cases occur in the UK each year

Prevalence is the total number of cases with a condition in a population at a particular point in time. It is affected by survival – prevalence will be closer to incidence in conditions with a short life expectancy, whereas prevalence and incidence will be more disparate in conditions with longer survival (such as PD). Prevalence is also affected by study methodology – estimates from hospital-based surveys produce lower figures than those derived from community-based studies. As a result of these

methodological difficulties, prevalence rates in PD vary widely between 18 (Shanghai, China) and 328/100,000 (Bombay, India). Less variation is seen if only UK-based studies are examined, which show prevalence rates of 108 to 164/100,000.

> Prevalence = number of cases in a population at a particular time. There are about 100,000 cases of PD in the UK at any one time

Both incidence and prevalence are markedly affected by the increase in PD with age. The age-specific incidence of PD rises exponentially into the 70s and 80s but then declines in most studies. This decrease is probably an artefact due to poor case ascertainment and the low numbers in these age groups. Age-specific prevalence also increases exponentially over the same age range.

> About 2% of the population >65 years has PD. Each primary care group has about 160 patients with PD and an additional 18 cases/annum are diagnosed

PD has been shown in studies to occur more commonly in males than in females. The average male:female ratio based on prevalence studies is 1.35:1, and from incidence studies 1.31:1. These figures are subject to considerable variation, probably due to the underlying age distribution of the populations examined, differences in survival, and access to healthcare.

Crude prevalence studies suggest that the occurrence of PD is more common in Caucasians in Europe and North America, intermediate in Oriental races in Japan and China, and lowest in African races. However, a door-to-door community study in North America showed similar prevalence rates in white and black populations. Thus, ascertainment bias may account for any apparent differences in prevalence between races.

It is impossible to ascertain whether or not there has been any change in the incidence or prevalence of PD over time; however, using the limited data available, adjusted for age and gender, Zhang and Roman have suggested no significant temporal change in either statistic over the past 50 years.

> The ageing population is expected to dramatically increase the number of cases of PD

Mortality

National mortality data

Although national mortality statistics are readily available, they are subject to the following confounding variables:

- accuracy of death certification, with the diagnosis of PD often omitted from certificates
- diagnostic difficulties between neurodegenerative conditions mimicking PD – these were compounded in the early part of the past century by cases of post-encephalitic parkinsonism
- changes in the way death certificate data are interpreted centrally

- changing age structure of the population.

Mortality data are most complete for England and Wales. Records date back to 1855, with a break between 1901 and 1920 when PD was not separately classified. The 300% rise in deaths between 1920 and 1989 was mainly due to the ageing population, but was also attributable to increased diagnostic accuracy. This increase continued into the 1990s (Figure 1.1). Age-specific mortality rates decreased in all age groups below 75 years from 1940 (Figure 1.2), which was probably due to the dying out of a cohort of patients with post-encephalitic parkinsonism (page 6). An increase in age-specific mortality in those over 75 years who presumably had PD was attributed to improved diagnosis.

The dip in mortality in the late 1970s and early 1980s was considered to be due to the introduction of levodopa (chapter 7). This was thought to delay the deaths of predominantly elderly parkinsonian patients for about five years, after which there was an increase back to expected levels as this group eventually died and added to the 'expected' deaths.

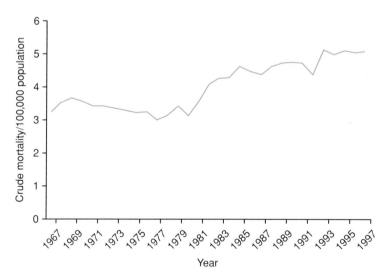

Figure 1.1
Crude mortality rate for PD in England and Wales. Data for 1984–93 have been corrected for changes in method coding death certificates. Reproduced with permission from Clarke CE. *J Neurol Neurosurg Psychiatry* 2000; **68**: 254–5

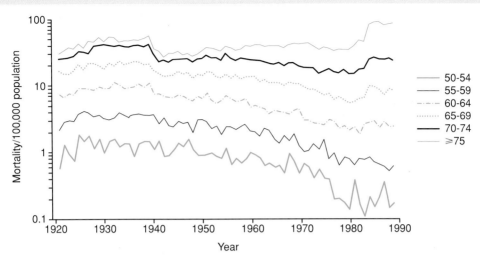

Figure 1.2
Age-specific mortality rates for PD in England and Wales. Reproduced with permission from Clarke CE. *J Neurol Neurosurg Psychiatry* 1993; **56**: 690–3

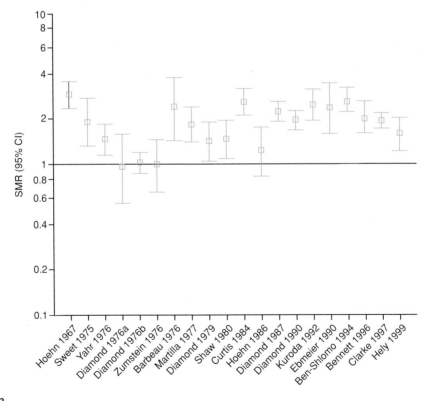

Figure 1.3
Standardized mortality ratios (SMRs) for cohort and case-control series examining mortality in PD plotted in chronological order of year of publication. Ratios >1 with 95% confidence intervals that do not overlap one indicate increased mortality in parkinsonian patients. Reproduced with permission from Clarke CE. *J Neurol Neurosurg Psychiatry* 2000; **68**: 254–5

Comparable trends in national mortality data have been reported from several Scandinavian countries and the US.

Cohort and case-control studies

Studies comparing the observed mortality in a group of PD patients with that expected from national mortality statistics are referred to as cohort studies. Case-control studies (page 5) examine mortality rates in two usually matched groups, one with and the another without PD, over the same time period. These study types in PD have been extensively reviewed (Figure 1.3). They show a fall in the ratio of number of deaths in PD patients to that in controls – the standardized mortality ratio (SMR) – in the early years of levodopa use (late 1970s and early 1980s) but a return to mean SMRs of 1.5 to 2.0 over the past decade. These studies show a statistically significant excess mortality rate, since the confidence intervals do not overlap one. In some, the upper 95% confidence interval overlaps the findings of the original Hoehn and Yahr study in the pre-levodopa era.

Thus, although the profound symptomatic impact of levodopa may not be disputed, its effects on mortality were short-lived. Cohort and case-control studies show that mortality from PD continues to be at levels comparable to those seen before levodopa was introduced.

These findings highlight the need for disease-modifying therapy as a matter of urgency.

> Mortality continues to be similar to that in the pre-levodopa era, although levodopa had a short-lived impact on mortality

Further reading

Ben-Shlomo Y. How far are we in understanding the cause of Parkinson's disease? *J Neurol Neurosurg Psychiatry* 1996; **61**: 4–16.

Clarke CE. Mortality from Parkinson's disease. *J Neurol Neurosurg Psychiatry* 2000; **68**: 254–5.

Clarke CE. Does levodopa therapy delay death in Parkinson's disease? A review of the evidence. *Mov Disord* 1995; **10**: 250–6.

Clarke CE. Mortality from Parkinson's disease in England and Wales 1921–89. *J Neurol Neurosurg Psychiatry* 1993; **56**: 690–3.

Hoehn MM, Yahr MD. Parkinsonism: onset, progression, and mortality. *Neurology* 1967; **17**: 427–42.

Schoenberg BS. Epidemiology of movement disorders. In: Marsden CD, Asbury AK, eds. *Movement disorders 2*. London: Butterworths, 1987: 17–32.

Schoenberg BS, Anderson DW, Haerer AF. Prevalence of Parkinson's disease in the biracial population of Copiah County, Mississippi. *Neurology* 1985; **35**: 841–5.

Tanner CM, Hubble JP, Chan P. Epidemiology and genetics of Parkinson's disease. In: Watts RL, Koller WC, eds. *Movement disorders: neurologic principles and practice*. New York: McGraw-Hill, 1997: 137–52.

Zhang ZX, Roman GC. Worldwide occurrence of Parkinson's disease: an updated review. *Neuroepidemiology* 1993; **12**: 195–208.

2. Aetiology

Environmental factors
Genetic factors

The cause or causes of idiopathic Parkinson's disease (PD) remain enigmatic. Time may prove that PD itself is more than one condition, each with more than one cause or perhaps with interacting causative factors. Several potential environmental and genetic factors may be associated with PD.

> There may be several types of idiopathic PD and each may have one or more causes

Environmental factors

Epidemiological studies in this area are comprised of:

- case-control studies, which examine in a group of PD patients and a matched control group the presence or absence of factors that may be causative for the condition. They may deal with present exposures (cross-sectional study) or those in the past (retrospective study)

- prospective studies, in which two groups of people, one exposed to and the other not exposed to a potential cause, are followed over time to assess how many develop PD.

Most PD studies are case-controlled and are, thus, likely to suffer from several potential sources of bias and other problems such as:

- differences in baseline characteristics of the patients and controls (eg age, sex)

- difficulty in later recall of low exposure to potential toxic agents in both cases and controls ('non-differential misclassification')

- high exposure to an agent may be better recalled by patients with PD ('recall bias')

- multiple significance testing may find associations by chance.

With these caveats in mind, a number of environmental factors have been shown to increase or decrease the risk of PD. These are summarized in Table 2.1 and are briefly discussed below.

MPTP, pesticides and farming

Interest in a potential neurotoxin as a causative factor for PD was re-kindled by the discovery that 1-methyl-4-phenyl-1,2,3,6-tetrahydropyridine (MPTP) caused a parkinsonian syndrome similar to PD (Figure 2.1). This was unwittingly synthesized in the

Table 2.1
Environmental factors associated with PD

	Increased risk	Decreased risk
Toxins	● Pesticides	● Cigarette smoking
	● Rural residence, farming, drinking well water	● Caffeine (coffee)
	● MPTP*	
	● Manganese, copper	
Infections	● Encephalitis lethargica	
	● Influenza	
Trauma	● Head injury	
Diet	● Vitamin supplements	

*MPTP=1-methyl-4-phenyl-1,2,3,6-tetrahydropyridine

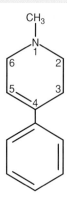

Figure 2.1
Chemical structure of MPTP

early 1980s by an enterprising chemistry graduate in San Fransisco, US, who had been creating his own pethidine (demerol)-analog for street sale. Intravenous drug abusers who received large doses of MPTP developed a profound parkinsonian syndrome, while about 400 with less exposure and no parkinsonian features are being followed long-term. Three of these patients recently died and autopsy revealed astrocytic and microglial infiltration with extraneuronal melanin in the substantia nigra, suggesting active neuronal loss. This implies that the toxin led to a progressive degenerative process and not a single toxic reaction.

MPTP is unlikely to be present in the environment in quantities sufficient to cause PD. It is, however, structurally similar to many other substances, including a number of pesticides. Several case-control studies have shown a small but significant increased risk of PD in those exposed to pesticides, rural residence, farming, and drinking well water. Some of this may, however, be attributable to recall bias. The introduction and increasing use of such agents has only occurred over the past three decades and no corresponding increase in the incidence of PD has been reported. The population's exposure to such agents is also relatively low, so it has limited significance in terms of public health.

Infections

The outbreak of post-encephalitic parkinsonism following the epidemic of encephalitis lethargica between 1917 and 1926 first raised the possibility that a virus may cause PD. Mortality data for England and Wales suggest that many younger cases of 'PD' in the past who have now died out were in fact due to subclinical encephalitis lethargica (page 2). Many other viruses have been proposed, but serological and autopsy support for such theories is lacking.

Head injury

James Parkinson first suggested that head injury may play a part in the genesis of PD. Although several studies have shown an increase in major and minor head injury in PD patients, this is an area where recall bias is particularly likely, so the results must be viewed with caution.

Vitamins

Vitamin supplements have also been associated with PD. Limited prospective data link vitamin E with an increased risk in women, and vitamin C with a reduced risk. Further confirmation is needed in longer prospective studies in both sexes.

Cigarette smoking

The paradoxical reduced risk of PD in cigarette smokers has been well established for many years from cohort and case-control series. There even appears to be a dose–response relationship. This association is also seen in young onset PD which excludes the 'competing cause mortality' explanation that smokers liable to PD die from smoking-related disease before they are old enough to manifest the movement disorder. Direct protective effects of smoking have been proposed to explain its beneficial effects but there is no evidence to support such a theory. It has also been suggested that a so-called 'parkinsonian personality' trait of introversion and caution may lead pre-symptomatic individuals to avoid novelty-seeking behaviours such as smoking.

> Cigarette smoking and drinking beverages containing caffeine are protective against PD for reasons that are unknown

Genetic factors

Family studies

Gowers, an English neurologist, drew attention to a familial predisposition to PD >100 years ago, but it was Mjones in 1949 who published the first large family study based on Swedish cases. Since then, many others have entered the debate with their own series, some concluding that PD is inherited by autosomal dominant inheritance with incomplete penetrance, a few suggesting polygenic inheritance, and others a multifactorial aetiology. A number of large kindreds with familial PD have been described in recent years. In most of these, an autosomal dominant pattern of inheritance was most likely. However, these families have features atypical of PD, such as early age of onset (third and fourth decades), and clinically multiple systems were affected.

Twin studies

The study of concordance rates in twin pairs offers a unique way to examine the genetic causation of a disease. A higher concordance rate (ie both twins having the condition) in monozygotic (identical) twins than in dizygotic (non-identical) twins strongly suggests a genetic aetiology. Initial twin studies in PD failed to find a higher concordance rate in monozygotic pairs. However, these studies examined only small numbers, introducing the possibility of a biased sample, and there remained the possibility that a second twin, unaffected at the time of the study, might have developed the condition in later years. The latter point was addressed in a study using positron emission tomography (PET) which demonstrated lower fluorodopa uptake and thus nigrostriatal neuronal loss in a number of

clinically unaffected twins, some of whom have gone on to develop PD – this suggested a higher concordance rate in monozygotic twins. The latest and largest contribution to this debate has been a study of 19,842 white male US World War II veterans. The concordance rate in 71 monozygotic twin pairs was 0.155 compared with 0.111 in 90 dizygotic pairs (relative risk 1.39; 95% CI 0.63–3.1). This non-significant result should be viewed with caution as it applies only to the male Caucasian population of the US; also, the study only evaluated subjects at one time point, without functional imaging, although they were older than 65 years at the time of screening. Interestingly, all four monozygotic twin pairs with a diagnosis before age 51 years were concordant, compared with only two of the 12 dizygotic twin pairs (relative risk 6.00; 95% CI 1.69–21.3). Although this statistically significant result is in keeping with the finding that large kindreds with autosomal dominant inheritance patterns tend to have a younger age of onset, the small numbers of twin pairs suggests that further work is required for confirmation.

> Monozygotic twins may have a higher concordance rate than dizygotic twins but this needs to be confirmed by further research

Candidate gene studies

In this approach, the genes potentially responsible for the biochemical abnormalities found in PD are examined in case-control series in the hope of finding linkage with the condition. This method has the benefit of allowing for multifactorial aetiology with gene-gene and gene-environment interactions. An example is the well-described defect in debrisoquine metabolism in PD due to deficient cytochrome P450 2D6 (CYP2D6) enzyme activity.

Genes for PD

The recent discovery of several genes for the condition was made possible by the use of molecular genetic approaches in screening large kindreds with familial PD (Table 2.2).

The first gene to be discovered was a single amino acid substitution in the gene for α synuclein in the large Italian-American Contursi kindred. This dominantly inherited form of parkinsonism was early in onset but was pathologically typical of the idiopathic condition. Although this mutation has been identified in other families, it appears to be a rare cause of familial PD. α synuclein is a highly conserved protein in nature, being upregulated in birds during song development. Its function in human neurones is unknown but it readily forms into β sheets and then aggregates, so the finding of α synuclein in Lewy bodies, the pathological hallmark of PD (chapter 3), may be a clue to the pathogenetic process.

> The α synuclein gene mutation accounts for a small number of familial cases

The next gene was discovered in Japanese families with autosomal recessive juvenile-onset disease. The Parkin gene codes for a protein with some similarity with ubiquitin. Ubiquitin is also a component of Lewy bodies but, intriguingly, these patients do not have Lewy bodies at autopsy. In another family, an abnormality in the gene for ubiquitin hydrolase L1 (UCH-L1) has been found associated with parkinsonism, although this requires further corroboration.

> The parkin gene accounts for a small number of young-onset (<40 years) cases

Mitochondrial inheritance

A deficiency of mitochondrial complex 1 has been found in PD, so it is conceivable that the condition may be transmitted through a mitochondrial gene defect. Since mitochondria are inherited through the maternal line, a maternal transmission pattern would thus be expected if this was the case. Although this has not been found in practice, this form of inheritance remains a possibility since most archetypal mitochondrial disorders, such as chronic progressive external ophthalmoplegia and the Kearns-Sayre syndrome, present as sporadic cases. It was recently found that the mitochondrial complex 1 deficiency in humans could be transmitted through isolated mitochondrial deoxyribonucleic acid (DNA) to so-called rho⁰ cells deficient in mitochondria. In the future, the hunt for a mitochondrial gene abnormality is likely to focus on sequencing the mitochondrial genome in patients with low complex 1 activity and a transmissible defect.

> PD may be transmitted through a mitochondrial gene defect, most probably through the maternal line

Table 2.2
Genes for PD

Name	Locus	Gene	Inheritance	Clinical features
Park 1	4q 21–23	α synuclein	AD	Mean age of onset 44 years
Park 2	6q 25.2–27	Parkin	AR	Juvenile-onset
Park 3	2p 13	?	AD	Late 50s and 60s onset
	4p 14	UCH-L1	AD	
	4p 14-	? (not UCH-L1)	AD	Onset in 40s; severe dementia
FTDP-17	17q 21-23	Tau	AD	Rapid progression; death in months

AD = autosomal dominant; AR = autosomal recessive; FTDP = frontotemporal dementia and parkinsonism; UCH-L1 = ubiquitin hydrolase L1

Further reading

Ben-Shlomo Y. The epidemiology of Parkinson's disease. In: Quinn NP, ed. *Parkinsonism*. London: Bailliere-Tindall, 1997: 55–68.

Ben-Shlomo Y. Smoking and neurodegenerative diseases. *Lancet* 1993; **342**: 1239.

Burn DJ, Mark MH, Playford ED *et al*. Parkinson's disease in twins studied with 18F-dopa and positron emission tomography. *Neurology* 1992; **42**: 1894–900.

Cerhan JR, Wallace RB, Folsom AR. Antioxidant intake and risk of Parkinson's disease in older women. *Amer J Epid* 1994; **139**: S65.

Gu M, Cooper JM, Taanman JW, Schapira AHV. Mitochondrial DNA transmission of the mitochondrial defect in Parkinson's disease. *Ann Neurol* 1998; **44**: 177–86.

Jarman P, Wood N. Parkinson's disease genetics comes of age. *BMJ* 1999; **318**: 1641–2.

Langston JW, Ballard PA, Tetrud JW, Irwin I. Chronic parkinsonism in humans due to a product of meperidine-analog synthesis. *Science* 1983; **219**: 979–80.

Langston JW, Forno LS, Tetrud J *et al*. Evidence for active nerve cell degeneration in the substantia nigra of humans years after 1-methyl-4-phenyl-1,2,3,6-tetrahydropyridine exposure. *Ann Neurol* 1999; **46**: 598–605.

Marsden CD. Twins and Parkinson's disease. *J Neurol Neurosurg Psychiatry* 1987; **50**: 105–6.

Nicholl DJ, Bennett P, Hiller L *et al*. A study of five candidate genes in Parkinson's disease and related neurodegenerative disorders. European Study Group on Atypical Parkinsonism. *Neurology* 1999; **53**: 1382–3.

Parkinson J. *An essay on the shaking palsy*. London: Sherwood, Neely, and Jones, 1817.

Piccini P, Burn DJ, Ceravolo R *et al*. The role of inheritance in sporadic Parkinson's disease: evidence from a longitudinal study of dopaminergic function in twins. *Ann Neurol* 1999; **45**: 577–82.

Riggs JE. Cigarette smoking and Parkinson's disease: the illusion of a neuroprotective effect. *Clin Neuropharmacol* 1992; **15**: 88–99.

Tanner CM, Hubble JP, Chan P. Epidemiology and genetics of Parkinson's disease. In: Watts RL, Koller WC, eds. *Movement disorders: neurologic principles and practice*. New York: McGraw-Hill, 1997: 137–52.

Tanner CM, Ottman R, Goldman SM *et al*. Parkinson's disease in twins: an aetiologic study. *JAMA* 1999; **281**: 341–6.

Ward CD, Duvoisin RC, Ince SE *et al*. Parkinson's disease in 65 pairs of twins and in a set of quadruplets. *Neurology* 1983; **33**: 815–24.

Wood N. Genetic aspects of parkinsonism. In: Quinn NP, ed. *Parkinsonism*. London: Bailiere-Tindall, 1997: 37–53.

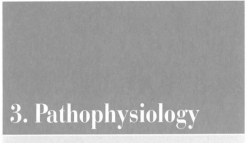

3. Pathophysiology

Neuropathology
Neurochemical abnormalities
Oxidative stress and free radicals
Functional anatomy of the basal ganglia

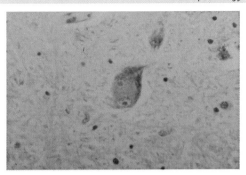

Figure 3.1
Typical brainstem Lewy body

Neuropathology

There are three pathological hallmarks of idiopathic Parkinson's disease (PD):

- the formation of Lewy bodies
- neuronal death in the pars compacta of the substantia nigra
- the removal of neuromelanin from dead cells by microglia.

Lewy bodies

Lewy bodies are eosinophilic intraneuronal inclusions named after the German pathologist. They are found in the catecholaminergic nuclei affected in PD, along with the cerebral cortex, thalamus, brainstem, intermediolateral column of the spinal cord, sympathetic ganglia, and myenteric plexus of the gastrointestinal tract. The classical nigral Lewy body (Figure 3.1) is composed of three layers:

- densely staining central core
- larger outer body
- surrounding halo.

In the cortex, the layers within the Lewy body are less distinct, but in the hypothalamus and sympathetic ganglia they may be multiple, may overlap and may even merge into elongated inclusions. Electron microscopy of a typical Lewy body reveals a sunflower appearance comprised of a body and a halo, which are composed of neurofilaments and a core made of granular material. The immunocytochemical staining characteristics of the granular material are complex but include phosphorylated neurofilaments, tubulin, microtubulin-associated protein (MAP) and ubiquitin. Ubiquitin is a highly conserved 76 amino acid protein that normally conjugates with other proteins to label them for non-lysosomal adenosine triphosphatase (ATP-ase)-dependent proteolysis. Anti-ubiquitin staining is particularly useful in identifying the rarer cortical Lewy body.

Although much information has been accumulated on the Lewy body, its precise role in the pathophysiology of PD remains unknown.

The prevalence of incidental Lewy bodies at autopsy in patients without signs of PD steadily rises from 4% in the seventh decade to 33% in the 11th decade. It is well established that clinical signs of PD do not develop until normal striatal dopamine levels are reduced by 80% and cell loss in the substantia nigra reaches 50%. This clearly suggests a pre-symptomatic phase of the illness and that those with incidental Lewy bodies at postmortem might have developed the condition had they lived. This evidence, coupled with the exponential rise in the prevalence of PD with age (chapter 1), raises important public health issues as the populations of developed nations age significantly over the next few decades.

4% of asymptomatic people in their seventh decade and 33% in their 11th decade will have Lewy bodies, suggesting a pre-symptomatic phase

Although the Lewy body is an essential feature in PD, it can also be seen in other conditions including Alzheimer's disease, Hallervorden-Spatz disease, multiple system atrophy (MSA) (chapter 4), progressive supranuclear palsy (PSP) (chapter 4), and the Parkinsonian-dementia complex of Guam. Presumably, it is a common endproduct of neuronal degeneration.

Neuronal death and neuromelanin removal

The loss of dopaminergic neurones from the substantia nigra pars compacta is an essential feature of PD. However, other catecholaminergic nuclei also suffer cell loss, including the ventral tegmental area, locus coeruleus, hypothalamus, raphé nuclei and sympathetic ganglia. The resulting loss of neuromelanin from the substantia nigra leads to the depigmentation of this structure at postmortem (Figure 3.2). The role of neuromelanin in the genesis of PD is unknown.

Neuronal death in the substantia nigra and Lewy bodies are the pathological hallmark of PD

Neurochemical abnormalities

The profound depletion of dopamine from the major output projection of the substantia nigra, the corpus striatum (caudate and putamen), was first reported by Ehringer and Hornykiewicz in 1960. This ultimately formed the rationale for the therapeutic breakthrough with the introduction of levodopa replacement therapy. Further work demonstrated similar dopamine depletion in the mesocorticolimbic and hypothalamic systems. The loss of 80% striatal dopamine before clinical features of PD develop suggests that good compensatory mechanisms exist. These consist of:

- a pre-synaptic increase in the turnover of dopamine in surviving neurones
- the postsynaptic increase in dopamine receptor sensitivity.

80% dopamine must be lost from the striatum before parkinsonian symptoms develop – the brain, therefore, has excellent compensatory mechanisms

The loss of neurones from the locus coeruleus in the brainstem leads to a depletion of cortical noradrenaline. Similarly, 5-hydroxytryptamine (5-HT) is reduced in the striatum due to raphé nucleus involvement.

Non-catecholaminergic neurones are also affected in PD. Loss of cholinergic neurones

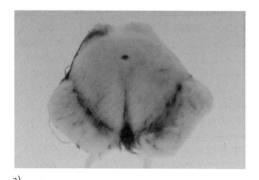

a)

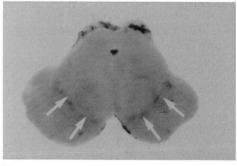

b)

Figure 3:2
Midbrain section from a) control and b) a patient with PD (arrows indicate depigmentation)

from the nucleus basalis of Meynert leads to reduced cholinergic innervation of the neocortex and hippocampus. Reductions in the peptides substance P, met-enkephalin, cholecystokinin and somatostatin in the basal ganglia in PD have been demonstrated, but the functional consequences of these changes are not known.

Oxidative stress and free radicals

Definitions

Oxidative stress occurs when there is excess production of free radicals. Free radicals are a series of molecules and chemical species that contain one or more unpaired electrons (Table 3.1). Electrons are usually paired and have opposite spins. With unpaired electrons, free radicals become highly reactive and oxidize agents by extracting electrons from other substances. This may result in damage to deoxyribonucleic acid (DNA), enzymes, other cellular proteins and unsaturated fatty acids. Natural defence mechanisms exist to destroy free radicals – enzymes such as superoxide dismutase (SOD) and glutathione peroxidase, and chemicals such as vitamin E, ascorbate, glutathione, urea compounds and ubiquinone can all scavenge and destroy free radicals.

Role in PD

A number of abnormalities in PD support the possibility that oxidative stress may play a part in the pathogenetic process. Glutathione levels in the nigra are reduced and some studies have shown reduced glutathione peroxidase activity. SOD levels are increased in both the cytosol

Table 3.1
Examples of free radical species

- Superoxide anion (O_2^-)
- Hydroxyl radical ($HO^•$)
- Nitric oxide (NO)
- Peroxynitrite ($ONOO^-$)
- Triplet oxygen ($^3O_2$)
- Singlet oxygen ($^1O_2$)

and mitochondria in PD nigral neurones, suggesting increased exposure to superoxide radicals. Polyunsaturated fatty acids, malondialdehyde and hydroperoxides – products of lipid membrane damage – are increased in PD nigra. In addition, 8-hydroxydeoxy-guanosine, a product of DNA damage, is increased in PD substantia nigra.

Iron can catalyse oxidative reactions that produce free radicals. Increased iron levels have been found in the substantia nigra in PD and may contribute to neuronal damage by increasing oxidative stress. A deficiency of 35% in respiratory chain complex I activity in mitochondria in PD may also predispose patients to oxidative stress.

> Oxidative stress, increased iron and deficient mitochondrial complex I are unclear in the pathogenesis of PD

Thus, multiple tantalizing pathological, neurochemical and biochemical abnormalities have been reported to occur in PD. At present, it is not known which of these is primary and which secondary, or even artefactual. Future work on abnormal gene products may allow a synthesis of these various abnormalities in familial cases of the disorder, which in turn is likely to help our understanding of sporadic cases (Figure 3.3).

Functional anatomy of the basal ganglia

Considerable strides have been made over the past 15 years in understanding the functional anatomy of the basal ganglia. The combination of neuroanatomical tracing studies, 2-deoxy-D-glucose autoradiography and microelectrode recordings have allowed a 'wiring diagram' of the basal ganglia to be assembled (Figure 3.4). As with any 'simple' explanation for a complex set of cerebral functions, this model has been found lacking in more recent years but still provides a detailed insight into certain aspects of PD physiology and has allowed a rational approach to novel surgical techniques in PD.

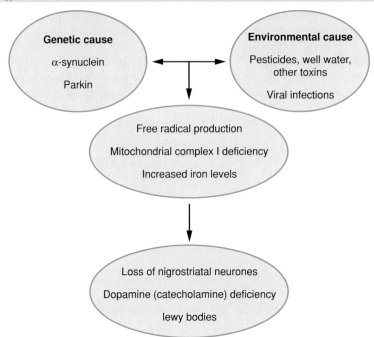

Figure 3.3
Postulated pathophysiology of PD

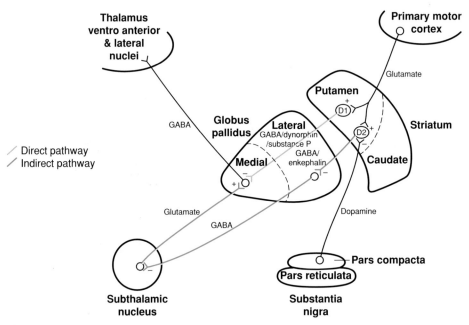

Figure 3.4
Major connections of the basal ganglia. + = excitatory neurotransmitter; − = inhibitory neurotransmitter

The pathway through the basal ganglia passes from the premotor cortex through the striatum and globus pallidus to the thalamus, and then back to the supplementary motor cortex. Activity in this loop is modulated by the substantia nigra which acts like a motor car accelerator, and the subthalamic nucleus (STN) which acts like a brake. In PD, the substantia nigra is defective and thus the accelerator fails to work and the patient slows down. Following a stroke (infarct) involving the STN, the brake is lost and the patient develops a contralateral hemiballismus/hemichorea syndrome.

> In normal conditions, the substantia nigra acts like a car accelerator on the basal ganglia, and the STN like a brake. Damage to the substantia nigra in PD slows the patient down, while damage to the STN speeds the patient up

On a more complex level, the functions of the nigra and STN are mediated through two pathways (Figure 3.4):

- ***direct pathway*** – this is comprised of gabaminergic neurones in the striatum projecting to the medial segment of the globus pallidus; these in turn inhibit gabaminergic neurones passing to the ventroanterior and ventroposterior nuclei of the thalamus. The inputs to this pathway are a glutamatergic projection from the premotor cortex and the nigral dopaminergic pathway

- ***indirect pathway*** – this is comprised of gabaminergic neurones in the striatum projecting to the lateral segment of the globus pallidus, which inhibit the gabaminergic neurones to the STN; these in turn inhibit the glutamatergic projection to the medial segment of the globus pallidum, which stimulates the gabaminergic neurones passing to the ventroanterior and ventroposterior nuclei of thalamus.

In PD, dopamine deficiency results in increased activity in striatopallidal gabaminergic fibres (Figure 3.5). This inhibits the lateral pallidal

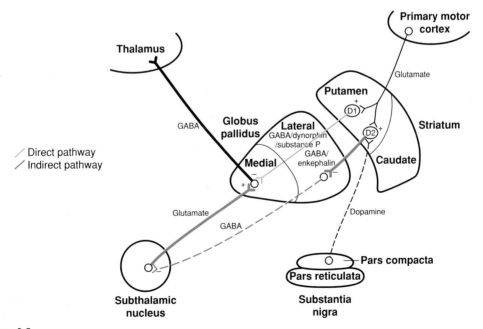

Figure 3.5
Changes in the basal ganglia in PD. Dotted lines represent decreased activity in pathway; solid lines represent increased activity in pathway; + = excitatory neurotransmitter; – = inhibitory neurotransmitter

gabaminergic neurones to the STN. The glutamatergic STN projection to the pallidum is thereby stimulated which increases the firing of medial pallidal gabaminergic neurones to the thalamus. Interestingly, these changes are the opposite to what happens in experimental models of chorea and ballism.

In levodopa-induced dyskinesia in PD, the opposite changes would be expected but this is not quite what is found. Instead of metabolic activity in the medial pallidum decreasing to normal with levodopa treatment, it increases. This could only be due to increased activity in the direct pathway from the striatum to the medial pallidal segment since the STN was inhibited. This leads to excessive inhibition of medial pallidal firing, as is seen in experimental models of chorea.

The above must be an oversimplification, since the peptides co-localized with GABA play no part in the model. Also, the somatotopic point-to-point projection of neurones is not taken into account, nor is the fact that each single line in the diagram represents around 10,000 individual neurones. However, it does explain why lesioning the STN (ie subthalamic nucleotomy) or switching off the STN (ie STN stimulation) in PD leads to improvement as the overactive subthalamopallidal glutamatergic pathway is disrupted. This is also the reasoning behind the search for glutamate antagonists for use in PD (eg remacemide).

> Overactivity in the glutamate pathway between the STN and medial segment of the globus pallidus in PD is central to new therapeutic strategies, ie STN lesions and stimulation

Further reading

Alexander GE, DeLong MR. Microstimulation of the primate neostriatum: II. Somatotopic organization of striatal microexcitable zones and their relation to neuronal response properties. *J Neurophysiol* 1985; **53**: 1433–46.

Crossman AR. Primate models of dyskinesia: the experimental approach to the study of basal ganglia-related involuntary movement disorders. *Neurosci* 1987; **21**: 1–40.

Ehringer H, Hornykiewicz O. Verteiling von noradrenalin und dopamin (3-hydroxytyramin) im gehirn des menschen und ihr verhalten bei erkrankungen des extrapyramidalen systems. *Klinische Wochenschrift* 1960; **38**: 1236–9.

Fearnley J, Lees AJ. Parkinson's disease: Neuropathology. In: Watts RL, Koller WC, eds. *Movement disorders: neurologic principles and practice*. New York: McGraw-Hill, 1997: 263–78.

Fearnley JM, Lees AJ. Ageing and Parkinson's disease: substantia nigra regional selectivity. *Brain* 1991; **114**: 2283–301.

Flaherty AW, Grabiel AM. Anatomy of the basal ganglia. In: Marsden CD, Fahn S, eds. *Movement disorders 3*. New York: Butterworth-Heinemann, 1994: 3–27.

Forno LS. Pathology of Parkinson's disease. In: Marsden CD, Fahn S, eds. *Movement disorders*. London: Butterworth Scientific, 1982: 25–40.

Jellinger K. The pathology of parkinsonism. In: Marsden CD, Fahn S, eds. *Movement disorders 2*. London: Butterworths, 1987: 124–65.

Mitchell IJ, Clarke CE, Boyce S et al. Neural mechanisms underlying parkinsonian symptoms based upon regional uptake of 2-deoxyglucose in monkeys exposed to 1-methyl-4-phenyl-1,2,3,6-tetrahydropyridine. *Neurosci* 1989; **32**: 213–26.

Mizuno Y, Ikebe SI, Hattori N et al. Aetiology of Parkinson's disease. In: Watts RL, Koller WC, eds. *Movement disorders: neurologic principles and practice*. New York: McGraw-Hill, 1997: 161–82.

Schapira AHV. Pathogenesis of Parkinson's disease. In: Quinn NP, ed. *Parkinsonism*. London: Bailliere-Tindall, 1997: 15–36.

4. Clinical features

Diagnostic signs and symptoms
Other features
Treatment-related complications
Differential diagnosis
Clinical rating scales

Diagnostic signs and symptoms

The cardinal diagnostic signs in early idiopathic Parkinson's disease (PD) are:

- hypokinesia and bradykinesia
- rigidity
- tremor at rest.

Hypokinesia and bradykinesia

Hypokinesia refers to the poverty of movement in PD. Patients lose facial expression and arm swing when walking. By contrast, bradykinesia refers to slowness of movement. The term akinesia implies no movement at all, but as this rarely occurs in PD the former two more precise terms are preferred although they are often imprecisely combined as bradykinesia. The difficulties generated by hypokinesia and bradykinesia cause the patient most difficulty with motor function.

Rigidity

The patient experiences this as a stiffness affecting all muscle groups, both axial and limb. On examination, rigidity is appreciated as a resistance to passive movement. When looking for rigidity, the clinician must always remember to re-inforce the movement by asking the patient to move the contralateral limb (Froment's sign). Thus, as the examined wrist is

flexed and extended, the patient should flex and extend the contralateral arm at the shoulder. That said, the pathophysiological basis of both rigidity and the effects of re-inforcement are not understood.

Extrapyramidal rigidity differs from spasticity – resistance to passive movement remains constant through the range of motion in extrapyramidal rigidity, while in spasticity there is a velocity-dependent increase in tone followed by relaxation which is called the clasp-knife phenomenon as it resembles the closure of a penknife.

Rigidity may feel smooth, so-called 'lead-pipe', or jerky due to superimposed tremor when it is referred to as 'cogwheeling'.

Tremor

Tremor is an involuntary rhythmical alternating movement. In PD, it is initially seen in one upper limb with intermittent opposition of the thumb and index finger, which is called 'pill rolling' tremor after the old method of making tablets. The frequency is typically 4–6 Hz. This spreads to the ipsilateral leg and then the other limbs as the condition progresses. Tremor is the first symptom of PD in about 75% of patients, but up to 20% of cases never develop tremor at any stage of the illness.

> Tremor is the first symptom of PD in ~75% of patients

It is important to specify the difference between parkinsonian tremor and essential tremor (ET) (page 21). Parkinsonian tremor occurs at rest while ET occurs when maintaining a posture (postural tremor) or performing an action (action tremor). Parkinsonian tremor is also clearly different from a cerebellar intention tremor, in which the amplitude of the tremor increases towards the point of intent. Inability to get the patient's limb at rest to observe a parkinsonian rest tremor is a common problem and is often best seen with the patient walking with both arms by his or her side. It has been known for many years that a postural tremor can be seen in PD in association with a rest tremor; however, it was recently found that this is often delayed in onset ('re-emergent'), unlike ET in which it begins as soon as the posture is adopted, and that it is of the same frequency as the rest tremor.

Precision of diagnosis

Studies from several brain banks in the early 1990s demonstrated that precision of the clinical diagnosis of PD was particularly poor. The United Kingdom Parkinson's Disease Society Brain Research Centre study of 100 consecutive patients with a clinical diagnosis of PD showed that only 76 had Lewy bodies in the brain at autopsy. Pedantic application of the previously reported diagnostic criteria (Table 4.1) only reduced this error from 24% to 18%. A recent study in north Wales has shown the diagnostic error rate of parkinsonian syndromes in general practice to be >50%. Since an accurate diagnosis has fundamental implications in terms of treatment response and prognosis, it is suggested that all patients with suspected PD are referred to a specialist with experience in diagnosing and treating the condition.

Postural instability

Postural instability is a fundamental feature of PD but, as it develops later in the course of the condition, it cannot be used as an early diagnostic feature. It is usually associated with a stooped posture with flexion of the cervical and thoracic spines. Imbalance is manifest as a tendency to fall either forwards or backwards. The slow shuffling gait at this stage of the condition combined with the postural difficulties leads to the forward 'festinating' gait and the propensity to shuffle and then to fall backwards, so-called 'retropulsion'.

Posture can be examined at the bedside by standing the patient with his or her feet slightly apart and then sharply pulling the patient backward (the 'pull test'). Falls represent a dangerous feature in later disease with the likelihood of fractures. If falls emerge

Table 4.1
United Kingdom Parkinson's Disease Society brain bank diagnostic criteria for PD

STEP 1 Diagnosis of parkinsonian syndrome
Bradykinesia (slowness of initiation of voluntary movement with progressive reduction in speed and amplitude of repetitive actions) and at least one of the following:

- muscular rigidity
- 4–6 Hz rest tremor
- postural instability not caused by primary visual, vestibular, cerebellar or proprioceptive dysfunction.

STEP 2 Exclusion criteria for PD
- History of repeated strokes with stepwise progression of parkinsonian features
- History of repeated head injury
- History of definite encephalitis
- Oculogyric crises
- Neuroleptic treatment at onset of symptoms
- >1 affected relative
- Sustained remission
- Strictly unilateral features after three years
- Supranuclear gaze palsy
- Cerebellar signs
- Early severe autonomic involvement
- Early severe dementia with disturbances of memory, language and praxis
- Babinski's sign
- Presence of a cerebral tumour or communicating hydrocephalus on computed tomography scan
- Negative response to large doses of levodopa (if malabsorption excluded)
- MPTP* exposure

STEP 3 Supportive prospective positive criteria for PD: three or more required for diagnosis of definite PD
- Unilateral onset
- Rest tremor present
- Progressive disorder
- Persistent asymmetry affecting the side of onset most
- Excellent (70–100%) response to levodopa
- Severe levodopa-induced chorea
- Levodopa response for ≥5 years
- Clinical course of ≥10 years

* 1-methyl-4-phenyl-1,2,3,6-tetrahydropyridine (page 5)

very early in the course of a parkinsonian syndrome, progressive supranuclear palsy (PSP) (page 22) is the more likely diagnosis.

> Hypokinesia and bradykinesia, rigidity and rest tremor are the diagnostic features of PD

Other features

Freezing

Freezing is the inability to initiate movement ('gait ignition failure') or the sudden stopping of movement when encountering an external stimulus such as a doorway. The neural mechanism of this intriguing symptom is unknown but it creates major difficulties for patients and does not respond to dopaminergic medication. Freezing should be differentiated from the sudden 'switching off' (immobile phase) that patients with levodopa-induced motor complications develop (chapter 7).

Paradoxical kinesia is the brief return of near normal mobility in PD in response to an urgent external stimulus such as an alarm bell.

Speech disorder

The speech disorder of PD is complex. The voice becomes monotonous and low in volume (hypophonia), with poor rhythm that can lead to repetition of the first syllable (palilalia).

Dysphagia

Dysphagia is seen later in the disease. It has been shown to respond to levodopa.

Excessive salivation

This is common in late PD but does not respond to antiparkinsonian therapy. Often, the best advice for patients is to chew sugar-free chewing gum which forces them to swallow.

Dystonia

Dystonia of the hand or foot can be seen in early untreated PD, but more commonly after levodopa therapy (chapter 7). Thus, writer's cramp can develop before other features of the disease. Calf cramp with or without obvious

dystonic plantar flexion and inversion of the ankle is common after treatment for some years. An unusual extension of the great toe ('striatal toe') can also be seen.

Frozen shoulder

Relative immobility and rigidity can lead to a frozen shoulder.

Oedema

Relative immobility and rigidity can also produce postural lower limb oedema.

Detrusor hyper-reflexia

Mild autonomic dysfunction is common in later PD, although this should be differentiated from the earlier and more profound autonomic problems seen in multiple system atrophy (MSA) (page 23). Detrusor hyper-reflexia leads to urinary frequency and urgency with, more rarely, incontinence in later PD.

Constipation

Constipation is almost universal in PD from the early stages of the illness.

Postural hypotension

Postural hypotension of a mild degree can be seen in later PD and can be exacerbated by levodopa and dopamine agonists.

Sleep disorders

Sleep disorders are common in PD (page 73). Some are due to other pathologies in this elderly population, such as prostatism. Others, such as vivid dreams and nightmares, are likely to be due to medication such as selegiline (chapter 6). Inability to turn over in bed is extremely common and is due to the deliberate use of short-acting medication, such as levodopa, during the day and not at night. Leg dystonia often occurs while the patient is in the 'off phase' in bed.

Restless Legs syndrome

The Restless Legs syndrome (RLS) is common in PD and can precede the condition by some years. It is comprised of irresistible leg movements, often accompanied by creeping sensations in the legs. The movements are worse with rest, particularly when trying to sleep. Effective treatment relies on levodopa or the dopamine agonists, suggesting that this condition is in some way related to dopaminergic deficiency.

Rapid Eye Movement (REM) Sleep Behaviour Disorder (RBD)

RBD has a rare association with PD. Normally during rapid eye movement (REM) sleep, we are atonic despite dreaming. In RBD, however, patients act out vivid dreams, sometimes in a violent fashion. Although RBD is not specific to PD, it can be the harbinger of the condition. Clonazepam 0.25–1.00 mg at night can reduce the symptoms of RBD but can give rise to excessive sedation or drowsiness.

Dementia

Dementia develops in about 20% of patients with later-stage PD. Typically, this gives rise to:

- poor, short-term memory
- fluctuating confusion
- visual hallucinations.

These problems become worse as a result of dopaminergic medication and can be precipitated by withdrawing the patient from the familiar environment of his or her home to respite care or hospital.

Dementia in PD can be difficult to differentiate from the more common Alzheimer's disease and multiple cerebral infarct dementia as all three can display parkinsonian signs. The value of an expert opinion from a clinician experienced in this diagnostic dilemma is inestimable. Some patients may present with dementia and no motor signs of PD but still have 'dementia with Lewy bodies'.

Depression

Depression is present in about 40% of patients with PD at any one time and is often overlooked. A recent quality of life study showed that it accounted for 40% of the

reduction in quality of life in PD compared with the 17% reduction caused by disease severity and medication.

Treatment-related complications

Although levodopa has a major beneficial effect in PD, it rapidly became clear after its introduction that it causes significant motor adverse events in long-term therapy (chapter 7). Thus, after five years of levodopa treatment, about 50% of patients will suffer from several motor complications. These and other complications of treatment in PD are outlined below.

Dyskinesia

Dyskinesia usually takes the form of involuntary athetoid movements of the limbs, trunk or face. These movements are worse in limbs most severely affected by PD itself. The neural mechanisms of dyskinesia still remain unclear.

Response fluctuations

Response fluctuations are comprised of:

- end-of-dose deterioration or 'wearing off' result in the effect of each dose of levodopa lasting for a shorter and shorter period. This contrasts with the effects of levodopa seen earlier in the disease, when sustained benefit is provided throughout the day
- unpredictable on/off fluctuations in which the patient switches rapidly and suddenly between the mobile so-called 'on' phase and the immobile 'off' phase, often as quickly as a light is switched on and off – this is not often appreciated by nurses or carers of the patient!

Response fluctuations are thought to be caused by progression of the underlying disease with further loss of nigrostriatal dopaminergic neurones and, thus, loss of the buffering capacity provided by the neurones' ability to store converted dopamine.

Dystonia

Although dystonia is a feature of PD itself, it is more common after levodopa therapy. The most frequently reported description is of early morning, 'off' period dystonia with painful calf cramps, and sometimes dystonic plantar flexion and inversion of the ankle. Paradoxically, this can be improved by taking the morning dose of levodopa. However, as levodopa initiates the problem, further escalation in dose will aggravate the dystonia. Its neural mechanisms are unclear.

Psychiatric complications

Psychiatric complications can be triggered by any of the treatments used in the later stages of PD. This, along with the observation of subsequent dementia in many such patients, suggests that the problems are due to a combination of the effects of medication and incipient Lewy body dementia. Psychiatric complications take the form of:

- hallucinations, often visual hallucinations of people or animals
- confusion, to the point that patients can no longer look after themselves independently
- a frank psychosis (very rare), which can develop with paranoid delusions.

> The main complications of treatment in PD are involuntary movements or dyskinesia, response fluctuations, dystonia and psychiatric problems

Differential diagnosis

The PD brain bank studies, that showed a 25% diagnostic error rate, were mostly performed on patients who had been diagnosed by a neurologist or geriatrician with an interest in PD. The diagnostic error rate is likely to be higher for those without such experience. It is often said that 50% of patients referred to movement disorder clinics with a diagnosis of PD do not have the condition – this is certainly my experience.

Essential tremor

The most common diagnostic error is believing that every patient with an isolated tremor has

PD – in fact, most of these patients will have ET. Recent work has suggested that ET is an autosomal dominant condition, the penetrance of which depends on age; thus, most affected individuals will have developed it by the time they have reached their 60s, if they live that long.

ET is a very common condition. Although prevalence studies in this area suffer from poor case-ascertainment, the prevalence of ET is likely to be in the region of 1,500/100,000 population (compared with PD at about 150/100,000). A general practitioner will, therefore, see about 10 times as many cases of ET as PD!

> ET is 10 times more common than PD, and it is often misdiagnosed as PD in general practice

Clinically, patients with ET most commonly present with a history of tremor of the upper limbs for a number of years, often more than five years. This contrasts with PD in which the tremor has usually been present for less than two years. The tremor occurs when maintaining a posture (ie holding the arms outstretched) and when performing an action (ie holding a teacup or screwdriver). The tremor of PD is mainly a rest tremor which disappears with posture and action. ET can affect the head, leading to titubation, and, rarely, the voice. It can be disabling in very few cases, which is the reason for recently dropping the epithet 'benign' from the title.

> ET usually comprises an upper limb postural tremor and an action tremor, lasting more than two years, whereas PD has a rest tremor presenting for less than two years

Treatment is confined to β-blockers (eg propranolol) and primidone, if tolerated, although botulinum toxin and functional neurosurgery are being explored for the more severe patients.

> ET may affect the head and voice

Presentation of a parkinsonian syndrome

For patients presenting with a parkinsonian syndrome of hypokinesia/bradykinesia and rigidity, with or without tremor, the differential diagnosis is much larger (Table 4.2).

Table 4.2
Differential diagnosis of a parkinsonian syndrome

- PD
- Drug-induced parkinsonism (by phenothiazines)
- Multiple cerebral infarct state
- Trauma – pugulistic encephalopathy
- Toxin-induced parkinsonism (by MPTP, carbon monoxide, manganese, copper)
- Parkinson's plus syndromes:
  - progressive supranuclear palsy (PSP)
  - multiple system atrophy (MSA)
    - Shy Drager syndrome
    - olivopontocerebellar atrophy
    - striatonigra degeneration

In practice, the rarest of these conditions can rapidly be dismissed after taking the patient's history and performing an examination using a checklist of 'red flags' (Table 4.3).

Table 4.3
Clinical features suggesting a parkinsonian syndrome is not due to PD

- History of severe cerebral trauma, stroke, exposure to neurotoxins or anti-dopaminergic agents
- Absence of rest tremor
- Symmetrical signs
- Associated ophthalmoplegia, pyramidal or cerebellar signs
- Associated autonomic dysfunction
- Rapid disease progression
- Poor response to levodopa

A group of Parkinson's plus syndromes initially appears so similar to PD that differentiation can be extremely difficult, even in experienced hands. Of these, progressive supranuclear palsy (PSP) and multiple system atrophy (MSA) are the two most common.

Progressive supranuclear palsy

PSP, or Steele-Richardson-Olszewski syndrome, typically presents with a symmetrical parkinsonian syndrome associated with early postural instability and falls, with the later development of a supranuclear ophthalmoplegia in which vertical, then horizontal eye movements are lost. Patients can develop:

- upper motor neurone signs in the limbs
- a pseudobulbar palsy with dysphagia and dysarthria
- upper motor neurone signs of slow spastic tongue movements
- a brisk jaw jerk.

Dementia is common in later stages of PSP

Pre-terminally, patients often suffer from a dementia. Rarer features can be useful in diagnosis, eg cervical dystonia leading to retrocollis (ie neck extension) and levator disinhibition which is a form of blepharospasm. The condition progresses more rapidly than PD and the parkinsonism is poorly responsive to levodopa. Pathologically, the condition is typified by the finding of neurofibrillary tangles and atrophy in the cerebral cortex, striatum, substantia nigra and brainstem. The tangles contain abnormally phosphorylated tau protein, which is a microtubular-associated protein involved in the axonal transport of vesicles.

PSP progresses faster than PD and does not respond as well to levodopa

---

Differentiating PSP from PD can be difficult as specific signs, mainly the eye movement disorder, are frequently absent within the first few years of diagnosis. The early postural instability and falls should lead to the suspicion of PSP. A patient with a parkinsonian syndrome who has falls in the first two or three years of developing the condition is likely to have PSP. Patients with PD tend to fall much later in course of the condition, after around eight to 10 years.

There is an early history of falls in PSP, and later supranuclear ophthalmoplegia with loss of downward and upward gaze and then horizontal movements

Multiple system atrophy

MSA is a relatively new term for a group of conditions that was previously thought to be unique. Recently, the similar terminal clinical features of these conditions and the discovery of a common glial cytoplasmic inclusion body have led to their unification under this specific heading.

Patients with MSA present in three broad categories, which loosely reflect the old nomenclature:

- Shy-Drager syndrome – present with autonomic dysfunction such as erectile failure, impotence, urinary incontinence and retention, faecal incontinence, postural hypotension and syncope
- olivopontocerebellar atrophy – present with cerebellar signs such as gait and limb ataxia and incoordination
- striatonigral degeneration – present with a relatively pure parkinsonian syndrome.

As the condition progresses, considerable overlap occurs in the clinical features and others such as upper motor neurone signs develop.

MSA presents with autonomic disturbance, cerebellar syndrome or parkinsonian syndrome, with an overlap in clinical features as the disease progresses

As with PSP, some rare but specific signs can be useful in diagnosis. These include:

- laryngeal dystonia leading to stridor and sleep apnoea, for which elective tracheostomy can be life-saving
- disproportionate antecollis, ie neck flexion with less kyphosis than is seen in PD

- stimulus-sensitive myoclonus, which is best elicited by a pin prick of the outstretched pronated hand.

The response to levodopa is poor in most patients but some can improve, especially with large doses, and a few may even develop dyskinesia, especially oro-facial. It is important to note that dementia *never* develops in MSA and is an exclusion criterion for the diagnosis. Disease progression is more rapid than in PD but slower than in PSP.

Dementia does not develop in MSA

Progression of MSA is faster than in PD and the response to levodopa is poor

As with PSP, differentiation of MSA from PD can be difficult in the initial stages when specific features are absent. Rapid progression and poor response to large doses of levodopa (about 1,000 mg levodopa with a decarboxylase inhibitor, eg Sinemet Plus 10 tablets daily) should alert the clinician to the possibility of MSA, especially in younger patients (with the mean age of onset being 54 years in MSA). Early autonomic features, such as impotence and urinary problems, strongly suggest MSA.

Specific features of MSA include laryngeal dystonia (stridor and sleep apnoea), disproportionate antecollis and stimulus-sensitive myoclonus

Drug-induced parkinsonism

Parkinsonism can be induced by various drugs. For example, patients given prochlorperazine to treat non-specific dizziness may develop a parkinsonian syndrome as a result of its anti-dopaminergic activity. The parkinsonism settles when such agents are withdrawn, but this can take months and occasionally years – some patients even require dopaminergic therapy.

Multiple cerebral infarct state

A multiple cerebral infarct state leading to 'arteriosclerotic pseudo-parkinsonism' is a common diagnostic problem, particularly in the secondary care setting. However, most of these patients present with a classical marche à petits pas gait (ie shuffling with small steps) with few, if any, signs of parkinsonism in the upper limbs. This is referred to as 'lower-half parkinsonism'. Such patients do not respond to levodopa and progress rapidly, usually developing other features of a multiple infarct state such as dementia, incontinence, transient ischaemic attacks and stroke. The only treatment is to attend to cerebrovascular risk factors such as hypertension, smoking, diabetes, etc. Computed tomography brain scanning may be necessary to exclude hydrocephalus in some cases.

Wilson's disease

This is an autosomal recessive condition with accumulation of copper within the liver leading to cirrhosis, and within the striatum leading to tremor, parkinsonism, chorea, and dystonia usually with some psychiatric features such as depression and personality change. It is, therefore, crucial in all young (<50 years) patients with parkinsonism to have serum caeruloplasmin and urine copper studies to exclude this disease.

Differential diagnosis, referral and treatment

Due to the considerable problems in accurately diagnosing the cause of a parkinsonian syndrome, even in expert hands, it is generally accepted that it is preferable for patients with suspected PD to be referred to a secondary care physician with a special interest in such movement disorders, before a firm diagnosis is made.

> Treatment for PD should not be initiated in the primary care setting without specialist advice

It is also best that such patients are referred before treatment is commenced because:

- they may not need treatment if they do not have PD
- treatment may mask the diagnosis of PD
- they may not have significant functional disability from their PD
- they may best be treated with dopamine agonist monotherapy if they are relatively young with PD.

> Primary care physicians should refer patients with suspected parkinsonism to a neurologist or geriatrician with an interest in PD for the most accurate diagnosis and the most appropriate treatment

Clinical rating scales

Primary care physicians do not require a working knowledge of the clinical rating scales used to measure the severity of PD, as these are only used in secondary care in the context of clinical trials. However, a summary of the Hoehn and Yahr scale (which is used to stage the patient's condition) is provided in Table 4.4 for those who wish to critically appraise such trials. Table 4.5 lists some of the more common scales used as outcome measures in trials.

Table 4.4
Hoehn and Yahr clinical rating scale

Stage of PD	Severity of PD
Stage 1.0	Unilateral involvement only
Stage 1.5	Unilateral and axial involvement
Stage 2.0	Bilateral involvement without impairment of balance
Stage 2.5	Mild bilateral involvement with recovery on retropulsion (pull) test
Stage 3.0	Mild to moderate bilateral involvement, some postural instability but physically independent
Stage 4.0	Severe disability, still able to walk and to stand unassisted
Stage 5.0	Wheelchair bound or bedridden unless aided

Table 4.5
Common outcome measures used in clinical trials in PD

Scale	Type of measure	Number of items
Investigator-rated motor scales		
Unified Parkinson's Disease Rating Scale (UPDRS)	Mentation (part I) – impairment	4
	Activities of daily living (part II) – disability	13
	Motor (part III) – impairment	14
	Complications of treatment (part IV) – impairment	11
	Modified Hoehn and Yahr – mixed	8
	Schwab and England – disability	20
	Total UPDRS score (total of parts I to IV above) – mixed	
Webster	Mixed impairment and disability	10
Northwestern University Disability Scale (NUDS)	Mixed impairment and disability	5
Patient on/off diary cards	Impairment	30 or 60 min epochs
Patient rated-quality of life scales		
Parkinson's Disease Questionnaire (PDQ) 39	Mixed impairment and disability	39
EuroQol EQ5	Mixed impairment and disability	5 and graticule
Short Form 36 (12)	Mixed impairment and disability	36 (12)

Further reading

Clarke CE, Gullaksen E, MacDonald S, Lowe F. Referral criteria for speech and language therapy assessment of dysphagia caused by idiopathic parkinson's disease. *Acta Neurol Scand* 1998; **97**: 27–35.

Cummings JL. Depression and Parkinson's disease: a review. *Am J Psychiat* 1992; **4**: 443–54.

Findley L, Peto V, Pugner K *et al*. The impact of Parkinson's disease on quality of life: results of a research survey in the UK. *Mov Disord* 2000; **15**(suppl 3): 179.

Gibb WRG, Lees AJ. The relevance of the Lewy body to the pathogenesis of idiopathic Parkinson's disease. *J Neurol Neurosurg Psychiatry* 1988; **51**: 745–52.

Golbe LI. Progressive supranuclear palsy. In: Watts RL, Koller WC, eds. *Movement disorders: neurologic principles and practice*. New York: McGraw-Hill, 1997: 279–95.

Hoehn MM, Yahr MD. Parkinsonism: onset, progression, and mortality. *Neurology* 1967; **17**: 427–42.

Hughes AJ, Daniel SE, Kilford L, Lees AJ. Accuracy of clinical diagnosis of idiopathic Parkinson's disease: a clinico-pathological study of 100 cases. *J Neurol Neurosurg Psychiatry* 1992; **55**: 181–4.

Jankovic J, Schwartz KS, Ondo W. Re-emergent tremor of Parkinson's disease. *J Neurol Neurosurg Psychiatry* 1999; **67**: 646–50.

Koller WC, Busenbark KL. Essential tremor. In: Watts RL, Koller WC, eds. *Movement disorders: neurologic principles and practice*. New York: McGraw-Hill, 1997: 365–85.

Lees AJ. The Steele-Richardson-Olszewski syndrome (progressive supranuclear palsy). In: Marsden CD, Fahn S, eds. *Movement disorders* 2. London: Butterworths, 1987: 272–87.

Lees AJ, Blackburn NA, Campbell VL. The nighttime problems of Parkinson's disease. *Clin Neuropharmacol* 1988; **11**: 512–9.

Lennox GG, Lowe JS. Dementia with Lewy bodies. In: Quinn NP, ed. *Parkinsonism*. London: Bailliere-Tindall, 1997: 147–66.

Litvan I. Progressive supranuclear palsy and corticobasal degeneration. In: Quinn NP, ed. *Parkinsonism*. London: Bailliere-Tindall, 1997: 167–85.

Quinn N. Multiple system atrophy – the nature of the beast. *J Neurol Neurosurg Psychiatry* 1989; **Suppl**: 78–89.

Quinn N. Multiple system atrophy. In: Marsden CD, Fahn S, eds. *Movement disorders* 3. Oxford: Butterworth-Heinemann, 1994: 262–81.

Schenck CH, Bundlie SR, Mahowald MW. Delayed emergence of a parkinsonian disorder in 38% of 29 older men initially diagnosed with idiopathic rapid eye movement sleep behaviour disorder. *Neurology* 1996; **46**: 388–93.

Wenning GK, Quinn NP. Multiple system atrophy. In: Quinn NP, ed. *Parkinsonism*. London: Bailliere-Tindall, 1997: 187–204.

5. Potential investigations

Neurochemical techniques
Neurophysiological techniques
Structural imaging
Functional imaging

The diagnosis of idiopathic Parkinson's disease (PD) can only be made on clinical grounds at present. In recent years, much effort has been made to try and develop a form of test for the condition, but to date this has largely been unsuccessful. However, many of the techniques briefly described in this chapter have led to a greater understanding of the pathophysiology of PD.

> There is no diagnostic test for PD – diagnosis relies on clinical judgment and is best made by a clinician with considerable experience in the condition

Judging a diagnostic test can be summarized as follows:

- Sensitivity = number with the condition and positive test (true positives) divided by number with the condition

- Specificity = number without the condition with negative test (true negatives) divided by number without the condition

- The 'best' tests have both high sensitivity and specificity (approaching 1.0)

- The best way to judge the balance between sensitivity and specificity is with receiver operator characteristics curves which guide the choice of test result 'cut-off'.

Neurochemical techniques

Acute apomorphine and levodopa challenge tests

The striking clinical response to levodopa and apomorphine, the subcutaneously administered dopamine agonist, in PD raised the possibility that acute challenges with these substances may be useful diagnostic tests for the condition. A systematic review of the small studies examining this issue located nine trials. These evaluated a group with a clinical diagnosis of PD ($n= 306$), and a group thought to have Parkinson's plus conditions such as multiple system atrophy (MSA) and progressive supranuclear palsy (PSP) (pages 22 and 23) ($n=130$). Acute challenge tests with levodopa, apomorphine or both were performed and the responses were monitored by several clinical tests using thresholds to define PD or non-PD. They were then compared with the diagnostic 'gold standard' – the response to chronic levodopa therapy over several months in the clinic. Although there were significant methodological problems related to defining the threshold levels, both acute challenge tests showed similar sensitivity and specificity in the diagnosis of PD as did chronic levodopa therapy (Figure 5.1). In addition, the heterogeneity tests in the meta-analyses and logistic regression analysis failed to show statistically significant variation between studies in the sensitivities or specificities. Since no significant difference was found between the acute tests and chronic levodopa therapy, there is no advantage in using the acute challenge tests as patients move on to have chronic levodopa therapy. Most will receive levodopa or a dopamine agonist. The value of the acute tests is, therefore, minimal.

The real challenge for these diagnostic tests is in very early PD when diagnostic uncertainty is at its peak. Systematic review of the four studies examining acute challenge tests in newly diagnosed, untreated PD patients ($n=209$) also reveals that these tests provide no advantage over chronic levodopa therapy (Figure 5.2).

(a)

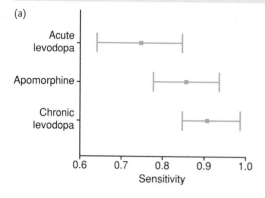

(b)

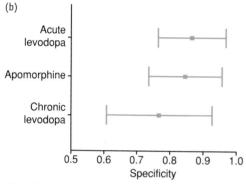

Figure 5.1
Meta-analysis of the (a) sensitivity and (b) specificity of acute challenge tests with apomorphine and levodopa therapy in the differentiation of PD from other Parkinson's plus conditions. Bars represent means and 95% confidence intervals. Reproduced with permission from Clarke, Davies. *J Neurol Neurosurg Psychiatry* 2000; **69**: 590–4

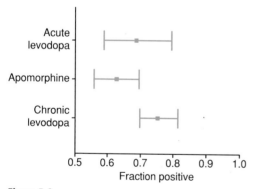

Figure 5.2
Meta-analysis of apomorphine, acute levodopa and chronic levodopa challenge tests in patients with newly diagnosed PD. Bars represent mean values and 95% confidence intervals. Reproduced with permission from Clarke, Davies. *J Neurol Neurosurg Psychiatry* 2000; **69**: 590–4

> Acute diagnostic tests with levodopa and apomorphine are of no additional value to chronic therapy with levodopa (and probably dopamine agonists)

Although acute apomorphine challenges may not be of any value in the diagnosis of PD, this does not preclude their use later in the disease either to demonstrate a continued response to dopaminergic therapy or as a prelude to apomorphine therapy.

Clonidine growth hormone stimulation test

Clonidine, the α_2-adrenoreceptor agonist, stimulates growth hormone secretion in healthy controls after intravenous injection by an action at the hypothalamic level. Reports of increased growth hormone secretion in response to clonidine in untreated patients with PD but not MSA raised the possibility that this may be a useful test for differentiating the two conditions. However, recent research has failed to replicate this work, possibly due to the considerable variability in growth hormone levels. More reliable tests of hypothalamic function may prove to be of value in this situation in the future.

Neurophysiological techniques
Anal sphincter electromyography

A small group of anterior horn cells in the sacral spinal cord, termed Onuf's nucleus, degenerates in MSA but not in PD. This leads to denervation of the external urethral and anal sphincters and thus causes the symptoms of bladder and bowel disturbance seen in MSA. The use of electromyography (EMG) of the urethral sphincter as a diagnostic test for MSA yielded a sensitivity of 0.62 and specificity of 0.92. Subsequent work using urethral sphincter EMG and/or the better-tolerated anal sphincter EMG has used different cut-off criteria but yielded similar results (0.74 and 0.89

sensitivity for MSA, respectively). However, denervation of the external anal sphincter has also been seen in five of 12 patients with PSP (sensitivity 0.42).

> Anal sphincter EMG is abnormal in MSA and some cases of PSP, but not in PD

It would be useful if confirmation of these results was available in a larger series of patients, as this would provide the opportunity to examine the diagnostic thresholds used in these tests with receiver operator characteristics curves. However, anal sphincter EMG is the only widely available investigation that can be used to differentiate PD from its mimics. Its main drawback is that it is an unpleasant procedure for the patient and, therefore, tends to be limited to those with clinical features suggestive of MSA.

Structural imaging
Computed tomography

The comparatively poor spatial resolution of computed tomography (CT) limits its value in the differential diagnosis of parkinsonian syndromes, although it can demonstrate brainstem and cerebellar atrophy in MSA. Its main use is in excluding other pathology in clinically atypical cases, such as a multiple cerebral infarct state, but the requirement for scanning should be the prerogative of the secondary care physician with experience in these conditions.

Magnetic resonance imaging

The superior resolution of magnetic resonance imaging (MRI) provides for more precise estimates of brainstem and cerebellar atrophy in MSA, and software developments now allow volumetric analysis of such structures. However, MRI has also demonstrated signal changes in some patients with MSA and PSP (Figure 5.3).

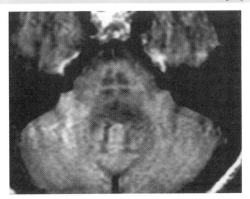

Figure 5.3
Proton density MRI in MSA showing increased signal in the brainstem (so-called 'hot-cross bun' sign). Reproduced from Watts RL, Koller WC. *Movement disorders: neurologic principles and practice*. New York: McGraw-Hill, 1997: 301.

Various combinations of atrophy and signal changes have been examined for their discriminatory value in the differential diagnosis of established parkinsonian syndromes. It has been concluded that an abnormal MRI is highly specific for MSA or PSP, whereas a normal MRI does not exclude the diagnosis because of the low sensitivity of the investigation. This low sensitivity hampers the value of MRI as a diagnostic test but has the advantage of being more readily available than most other modalities considered in this chapter.

> MRI abnormalities are specific for MSA and PSP but a normal test does not exclude them

Functional imaging
Magnetic resonance spectroscopy

Proton magnetic resonance spectroscopy (MRS) can provide information on the concentrations of intermediary metabolites in a small volume of cerebral tissue. The metabolite of largest concentration is N-acetylaspartate (NAA), which is found principally in neurones and their processes. The creatine (Cr) peak is taken as a marker of energy status and that for choline

(Cho) as an indicator of membrane synthesis and degradation. Additional smaller peaks can be seen at short echo times representing glutamate, aspartate and inositol. Review of MRS studies in parkinsonian syndromes demonstrates considerable heterogeneity in the results which preclude any firm conclusions being reached at present. Further large multicentre trials are required, preferably using absolute quantitation of tissue metabolite concentrations.

Positron emission tomography

In positron emission tomography (PET), a positron-emitting radioactive isotope is tagged to a molecule of interest or tracer which is then administered to the patient, usually by intravenous injection. This is taken up by the area of interest. The isotope then emits positrons which annihilate with electrons producing two high-energy γ-rays at 180° to one another. Coincidental hits by the γ-rays at two opposing sodium iodide detectors can be registered allowing measurement of absolute

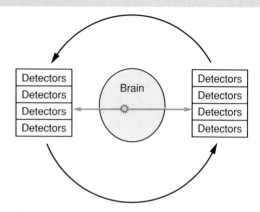

Figure 5.4
Principle of positron emission tomography. Green arrows represent release of two γ-rays at 180° to each other

tissue concentration of the isotope and thus of the molecule of interest (Figure 5.4). This can be processed to produce traditional two-dimensional images (tomographs) and more recently three-dimensional parametric maps of tracer uptake.

Table 5.1
PET and single photo emission tomography (SPECT) tracers and their uses in studying parkinsononian syndromes

Biological application	Tracer
Blood flow	$H_2{}^{15}O$, ^{99m}Tc-HMPAO, ^{133}Xe
Oxygen metabolism	$^{15}O_2$
Glucose metabolism	^{18}F-2-fluoro-2-deoxyglucose (^{18}FDG)
Dopamine storage	^{18}F-6-fluorodopa (^{18}F-dopa)
Dopamine vesicle transporters	^{11}C-dihydrotetrabenazine (DHTBZ)
Dopamine re-uptake sites	^{11}C-CFT, ^{11}C-RTI-32, ^{11}C-RTI-121
	^{11}C-nomifensine
	^{123}I-β-CIT, ^{123}I-FP-CIT, ^{123}I-IPT
Dopamine D_1 sites	^{11}C-SCH 23390
Dopamine $D_{2/3}$ sites	^{11}C-raclopride
	^{11}C-methylspiperone (MSP)
	^{18}F-fluoroethylspiperone
	^{76}Br-bromospiperone (BSP)
	^{123}I-iodobenzamide (IBZM)
	^{123}I-epidipride
MAO* B activity	^{11}C-deprenyl
Opioid binding	^{11}C-diprenorphine

* monoamine oxidase

PET tracers

Table 5.1 shows the tracers used and their applications. The drawbacks of this technique are:

- its expense
- the need to manufacture the isotopes immediately before injection using a cyclotron.

As a result, there are few PET scanners available.

The most valuable PET tracer in PD work has proved to be ^{18}F-6-fluorodopa (^{18}F-dopa). This is taken up by the nigrostriatal dopaminergic neurones and is converted into ^{18}F-dopamine and its metabolites. The rate of accumulation of ^{18}F is dependent on the transport of ^{18}F-dopa into the brain, neurones and then vesicles, versus its rate of breakdown. ^{18}F-dopa PET was first examined in PD in the early 1980s. Uptake was reduced by about 30% at the onset of the disease (Figure 5.5). This compares with the $\geq$80% loss of dopamine and dopaminergic neurones which highlights the compensatory mechanisms available in the striatum. In twin studies, ^{18}F-dopa PET has identified pre-clinical PD in apparently unaffected co-twins. Fascinating follow-up ^{18}F-dopa PET studies in PD have shown an annual decline in uptake of about 9–12%. This suggests a pre-clinical period of three to six years which is in keeping with data on the rate of nigral cell loss. This finding produces a window for neuroprotective therapies provided potential patients can be identified at this pre-clinical stage. ^{18}F-dopa PET is currently being used to assess whether or not potential neuroprotective therapies are effective and it has already demonstrated that fetal dopaminergic transplants can survive in PD.

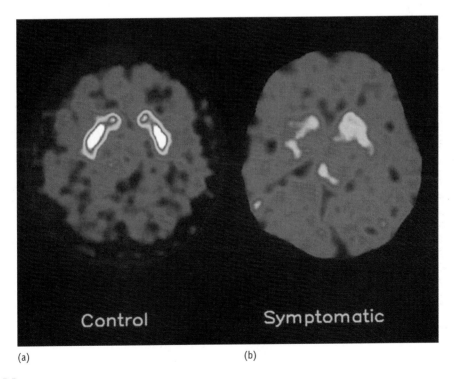

(a)　　　　　　　　　　　　　(b)

Figure 5.5
Fluorodopa PET uptake in (a) a control subject and (b) a patient with PD. Reproduced with permission from Watts RL, Koller WC. *Movement disorders: neurologic principles and practice.* New York: McGraw-Hill, 1997

[18]F-dopa PET plays no part in the differential diagnosis of parkinsonian syndromes as its uptake is also reduced in some patients with MSA and discriminant analysis cannot separate the two groups.

Various PET tracers have been used to examine postsynaptic dopamine receptors in parkinsonian disorders and the findings are summarized in Table 5.2.

Single photon emission tomography (SPECT)

SPECT follows similar principles to PET but uses more readily produced isotopes (eg [99m]technicium, [123]iodine) and consequently different tracers (Table 5.1). The result is a more practical and less expensive tool but at the expense of spatial resolution.

The labelled cocaine derivatives ^{123}I-β-CIT and ^{123}I-FP-CIT have most commonly been used with SPECT to label the pre-synaptic dopamine reuptake site and, thus, the pre-synaptic neurone, rather like ^{18}F-dopa in PET scanning. ^{123}I-FP-CIT has faster kinetics so that patients can be scanned several hours after injection instead of returning the next day as with ^{123}I-β-CIT (Figure 5.6). Both show a substantial fall in early PD but also in MSA. However, they can be useful in discriminating PD from essential tremor (ET) (page 21) in more difficult cases.

> PET and SPECT identify dopaminergic neurone loss but cannot reliably differentiate PD, MSA and PSP

Table 5.2

Summary of the changes seen with PET in dopamine receptors in PD

Receptor	Untreated		Treated	
	Putamen	Caudate	Putamen	Caudate
D_2	Normal or increased	Normal	Normal or decreased	Normal or decreased
D_1	Normal	Normal	Decreased	Decreased

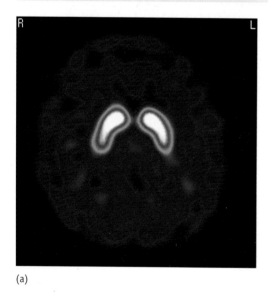
(a)

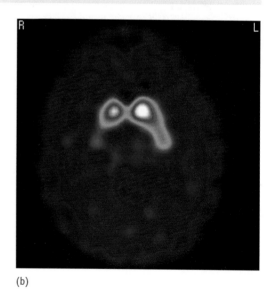
(b)

Figure 5.6
FP-CIT SPECT scans of (a) a control subject and (b) a patient with PD. Sourced from Dr H Benamer

Further reading

Booij J, Tissingh G, Winogrodzka A, van Royen EA. Imaging of the dopaminergic neurotransmission system using single photon emission tomography in patients with Parkinsonism. *Eur J Nuc Med* 1999; **26:** 171–82.

Brooks DJ. PET and SPECT studies in Parkinson's disease. In: Quinn NP, ed. *Parkinsonism*. London: Bailliere Tindall, 1997: 69–87.

Burn DJ, Mark MH, Playford ED *et al*. Parkinson's disease in twins studied with ^{18}F-dopa and positron emission tomography. *Neurology* 1992; **42:** 1894–900.

Burn DJ, Sawle GV, Brooks DJ. Differential diagnosis of Parkinson's disease, multiple system atrophy, and Steele-Richardson-Olszewski syndrome: discriminant analysis of striatal 18F-dopa PET. *J Neurol Neurosurg Psychiatry* 1994; **57:** 278–84.

Clarke CE, Davies P. Systematic review of acute levodopa and apomorphine challenge tests in the diagnosis of idiopathic Parkinson's disease. *J Neurol Neurosurg Psychiatry* 2000; **69:** 590–4.

Clarke CE, Ray PS, Speller JM. Failure of the clonidine growth hormone stimulation test to differentiate Multiple System Atrophy from advanced idiopathic Parkinson's disease. *Lancet* 1999; **353:** 1329–30.

Eardley I, Quinn NP, Fowler CJ *et al*. The value of urethral sphincter electromyography in the differential diagnosis of parkinsonism. *Brit J Urol* 1989; **64:** 360–2.

Fearnley JM, Lees AJ. Ageing and Parkinson's disease: substantia nigra regional selectivity. *Brain* 1991; **114:** 2283–301.

Kimber JR, Watson L, Mathias CJ. Distinction of idiopathic Parkinson's disease from multiple-system atrophy by stimulation of growth-hormone release with clonidine. *Lancet* 1997; **349:** 1877–81.

Kraft E, Schwarz J, Trenkwalder C *et al*. The combination of hypointense and hyperintense signal changes in T2-weighted magnetic resonance imaging sequences. A specific marker for multiple system atrophy? *Arch Neurol* 1999; **56:** 225–8.

Morrish PK, Rakshi JS, Bailey DL *et al*. Measuring the rate of progression and estimating the preclinical period of Parkinson's disease with [18F] dopa PET. *J Neurol Neurosurg Psychiatry* 1998; **64:** 314–9.

Morrish PK, Sawle GV, Brooks DJ. An 18F-dopa PET and clinical study of the rate of progression in Parkinson's disease. *Brain* 1996; **119:** 585–91.

Morrish PK, Sawle GV, Brooks DJ. Clinical and [18F] dopa PET findings in early Parkinson's disease. *J Neurol Neurosurg Psychiatry* 1995; **59:** 597–600.

Pramstaller PP, Wenning GK, Smith SJM *et al*. Nerve conduction studies, skeletal muscle EMG, and sphincter EMG in multiple system atrophy. *J Neurol Neurosurg Psychiatry* 1995; **58:** 618–21.

Schrag A, Kingsley D, Phatouros C *et al*. Clinical usefulness of magnetic resonance imaging in multiple system atrophy. *J Neurol Neurosurg Psychiatry* 1998; **65:** 65–71.

Schulz JB, Skalej M, Wedekind D *et al*. Magnetic resonance imaging-based volumetry differentiates idiopathic Parkinson's disease from multiple system atrophy and progressive supranuclear palsy. *Ann Neurol* 1999; **45:** 65–74.

Stocchi F, Carbone A, Inghilleri M *et al*. Urodynamic and neurophysiological evaluation in Parkinson's disease and multiple system atrophy. *J Neurol Neurosurg Psychiatry* 1997; **62:** 507–11.

Thomaides TN, Chaudhuri KR, Maule S *et al*. Growth hormone response to clonidine in central and peripheral primary autonomic failure. *Lancet* 1992; **340:** 263–6.

Tranchant C, Guiraud-Chaumeil C, Warter JM. Stimulation of growth hormone release with clonidine is not a good test to distinguish Parkinson's disease from multiple system atrophy. *Mov Disord* 1998; **13**(suppl 2): 197.

Valldeoriola F, Valls-Sole J, Tolosa ES, Marti MJ. Striated anal sphincter denervation in patients with progressive supranuclear palsy. *Mov Disord* 1995; **10:** 550–5.

6. Medical management – neuroprotection

Selegiline
Other potential neuroprotective strategies

Idiopathic Parkinson's disease (PD) is a steadily progressive condition. At present, pharmacotherapy can only provide symptomatic benefit to patients. What is required is an agent that can slow the progression of the disease – so-called neuroprotective therapy – or something that can permanently prevent the death of sick nigrostriatal dopaminergic neurones – so-called neurorescue therapy (Figure 6.1).

> No agent can be used to slow the disease progression of PD

The only potential neuroprotective therapy to be examined in any detail has been selegiline and, after many clinical trials, the debate continues as to whether it is protective or even harmful.

Selegiline

Brief history

Selegiline is a monoamine oxidase (MAO) inhibitor. This class of drug was developed in the 1950s after the serendipitous discovery that iproniazid, an early anti-tuberculous agent, had an antidepressant action that was related to MAO inhibition. Limited trials of MAO inhibitors in PD in the early 1960s, soon after the discovery of levodopa therapy, were disappointing because of the potentially dangerous increase in catecholamines producing the 'cheese reaction'. In 1968, however, two types of MAO inhibitors were determined, and it was found that the MAO B inhibitors were free from the cheese reaction. The MAO B inhibitor selegiline (synonymous in the US with deprenyl) was developed in the mid-1970s and was soon shown to have mild symptomatic benefits in PD.

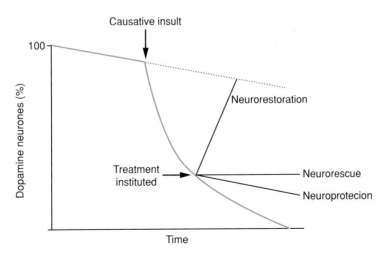

Figure 6.1
Schematic representation of neuroprotection, neurorescue, and neurorestoration in PD therapy

Mode of action

The main action of selegiline is to block MAO B, both in neurones and in glial cells. This reduces the degradation of dopamine (Figure 7.3, page 48) and thus increases the amount available at the synaptic cleft. However, selegiline is broken down into a number of metabolites including amphetamine and methamphetamine. The latter may be active and partly responsible for some of the actions of the drug. Selegiline metabolites are also likely to cause some of its adverse effects, such as sleep disturbance, vivid dreams and nightmares, which are discussed in chapter 9.

> Selegiline acts by inhibiting MAO B, which reduces dopamine degradation

Clinical studies

The interest in selegiline as a neuroprotective agent stemmed from the discovery in the early 1980s that it impaired the metabolism of 1-methyl-4-phenyl-1,2,3,6-tetrahydropyridine (MPTP) (page 5) into its active metabolite, the 1-methyl-4-phenyl-pyridine ion (MPP+), in experimental models of parkinsonism. Around the same time, it was found that selegiline could reduce the formation of a number of free radicals in vitro. There then appeared a retrospective longitudinal clinical study in PD from Birkmayer and colleagues in 1985. This was a non-randomized, open-label study which involved 377 patients who had received Madopar (levodopa/benserazide) alone and 564 who had received Madopar and selegiline over a mean follow-up period of nine years. Survival analysis demonstrated significantly improved survival in those given selegiline (mean survival Madopar alone 129 months v Madopar and selegiline 145 months; $p<0.001$). This study has been criticized for being retrospective and non-randomized.

DATATOP study

A small prospective double-blind study was later performed by Tetrud and Langston involving 54 patients with untreated PD, which showed that selegiline delayed the need for levodopa. It was clear that a large prospective study was required to examine the effect of selegiline on the course of PD. Thus, the North American Deprenyl and Tocopherol Antioxidative Therapy of Parkinsonism (DATATOP) study was designed under the auspices of the Parkinson Study Group. This study randomized 800 previously untreated patients with PD to receive blinded therapy with placebos, selegiline (deprenyl 10 mg/day), tocopherol (the biologically active component of vitamin E), or both drugs. After 12 months, 97 patients on selegiline reached the endpoint of requiring levodopa compared with 176 patients not taking selegiline (hazard ratio 0.43; 0.33, 0.55 95% CI; $p<10^{-10}$); tocopherol had no effect. It was concluded that selegiline could and should be used to delay levodopa therapy, but the question of whether or not the action of selegiline was purely symptomatic or neuroprotective could not be answered from this interim analysis.

> Selegiline can be used to delay the need for levodopa, but there is no clear evidence that it is neuroprotective

Patients in the DATATOP study who had not reached the endpoint were withdrawn from experimental treatment and followed over the next two months before all were treated with open-label selegiline. In these patients, a clear benefit on commencing selegiline was seen in Unified Parkinson's Disease Rating Scale (UPDRS) motor score and a similar deterioration when it was withdrawn. Again, any benefit from selegiline could have been due to its symptomatic effects rather than neuroprotection.

Examination of motor complications in patients who went on to use levodopa early in the trial showed that they occurred with a similar frequency in the selegiline-treated and untreated patients. Of those who did not go on to levodopa early but received open-label selegiline when the study design was changed, progression to needing levodopa occurred faster in patients who had previously been randomized to selegiline, suggesting that the initial advantages of selegiline were not maintained.

Mortality rates have also been documented after a mean of 8.2 years of observation. No differences between the treatment groups were found, although it should be noted that all patients received open-label selegiline for about three-and-a-half years after a mean period on double-blind medication of around three years. Table 6.1 summarizes the main findings of the DATATOP study.

SINDAPAR study

A further North American two-centre study (the SINDAPAR study) randomized 101 untreated PD patients to selegiline and Sinemet (levodopa/carbidopa), placebo and Sinemet, selegiline and bromocriptine, or placebo and bromocriptine. After a 12-month follow-up period, selegiline once again delayed the progression in UPDRS motor and activities of daily living (ADL) scores but after two months wash out of the selegiline or placebo, there was no significant difference between treatment groups in the deterioration in UPDRS scores; this was against a neuroprotective effect. In a small subset of 23 patients, the Sinemet or bromocriptine was also withdrawn for 14 days. There was less deterioration from baseline UPDRS scores for

those randomized to selegiline which was statistically significant, even though the sample size in this subgroup analysis was very small. This favoured a neuroprotective effect although the small numbers and the relatively short withdrawal period suggest this needs further confirmation.

UK PDRG study

Another large but open-label trial of selegiline therapy has been performed in the UK by the Parkinson's Disease Research Group (PDRG). This study involved 782 patients who were randomized to receive Madopar, Madopar and selegiline, or bromocriptine. After a mean of three years follow-up, motor impairment was similar in the two levodopa-treated groups but with more adverse events in the selegiline arm. The bromocriptine-treated patients were worse in terms of motor impairments but had fewer motor complications. It was concluded that the choice of first-line therapy in early disease may not be critical.

The bombshell came with the next interim analysis of this trial after a mean period of observation of 5.6 years. The mortality rate, adjusted for all baseline factors, was greater in the Madopar/selegiline-treated group than in the Madopar alone group (hazard ratio 1.57; 1.07, 2.31 95% CI). Motor impairment was similar in both groups but motor complications were worse with selegiline. As a result, all patients in the trial were withdrawn from selegiline.

Since this increase in mortality with selegiline had not previously been observed, a careful blinded assessment of patient case notes and death certificates was undertaken. This extended the follow up period to 6.8 years when the excess mortality in the selegiline group, corrected for baseline factors, was 1.30 (0.99, 1.72 95% CI) which is technically not significant since the lower confidence interval overlaps unity. The only differences found in clinical characteristics were an increased likelihood of dementia and a history of falls

---

Table 6.1
Summary of the main findings of the DATATOP study

- Selegiline delayed the need for levodopa by about nine months
- Whether or not the effect of selegiline was due to a symptomatic or a neuroprotective effect remains unclear
- Motor complications developed at the same rate in those initially treated with selegiline
- Mortality was not shown to be improved in those initially treated with selegiline
- Tocopherol (vitamin E) was ineffective

---

before death in the selegiline-treated patients. The key points relating to the PDRG trial are summarized in Table 6.2.

> The increased mortality in the selegiline arm of the UK PDRG study was not statistically significant when corrected for baseline covariants – this has not been shown in any other trial with this drug

There followed a furious debate in the correspondence columns of a number of general and neurology journals regarding the findings of the PDRG. This centred around:

- the increased mortality being 'out-of-step' with the DATATOP results and other smaller selegiline trials
- open-label studies being unreliable because of performance bias
- the trial being stopped on a random high in mortality
- the mortality being high in both groups
- the large number of patients who had switched medication
- the use of a significance level of just $p<0.05$ with several interim analyses of mortality in a 10-year study.

Unfortunately, the only systematic review and meta-analysis of early selegiline therapy trials failed to include all of the relevant studies and

Table 6.2

Summary of the main findings of the PDRG study

- Patients treated with selegiline showed increased mortality, although this was not significant when baseline covariants were accounted for
- No reason for increased mortality in the selegiline-treated patients could be found but there was a trend towards a link with dementia and a history of falls
- There were more adverse events in the selegiline arm
- Patients receiving bromocriptine monotherapy had worse motor impairment scores and a high dropout rate

the Cochrane reviews of selegiline are eagerly awaited.

Study of the UK General Practice Research Database

More recently, a study of the UK General Practice Research Database has been undertaken which included 12,621 patients aged 35–90 years who received a prescription for an antiparkinsonian drug between 1987 and 1996. There was a non-significant increase in mortality in those who had been given selegiline alone or in combination with levodopa (hazard ratio corrected for baseline factors 1.11; 1.00, 1.23 95% CI).

Why selegiline might increase mortality remains unresolved. However, two studies have now shown that selegiline can produce orthostatic hypotension which at times can be severe. This might increase the likelihood of stroke and myocardial infarction and thus death.

More recent trials

The latest five-year trial of selegiline combined with levodopa versus levodopa alone in PD ($n=163$) showed less deterioration in motor function in those given selegiline. Motor function did not deteriorate on selegiline washout over one month, suggesting that the beneficial effects were not due to a symptomatic effect but perhaps neuroprotection.

While this debate raged, clinicians in the UK who had previously acted on the assumption that selegiline might be neuroprotective and used it in most patients, changed their view. With the possibility of increased mortality, they were not prepared to take any risks and so withdrew selegiline from many or most of their patients. Thus, prescription rates fell in the UK by about two-thirds (Figure 6.2).

Even with a careful systematic review and meta-analysis of the mortality data from the selegiline trials, it is unlikely that any definitive conclusion can be reached. Further trial data are required from large numbers of

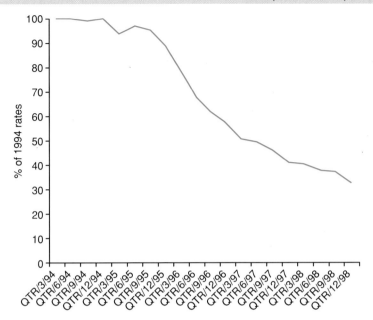

Figure 6.2
Standardized selegiline prescription rates in the UK. Reproduced with permission from IMS Health (Medical Data Index)

patients. These may emerge from the large pragmatic trial PD MED which is based in the University of Birmingham Clinical Trials Unit, Birmingham, and funded by the Health Technology Assessment Programme of the NHS Research and Development Programme. This will randomize untreated PD patients to any levodopa preparation, dopamine agonist or selegiline preparation, and will follow patients for 10 years using quality of life, health economics assessment and mortality as the main outcome measures.

The novel Zelapar selegiline preparation has recently been introduced. This is rapidly absorbed after application to the tongue as it is contained within a fast melt matrix. It is absorbed pre-gastrically and therefore does not undergo the extensive first-pass metabolism of orally administered selegiline (data on file with manufacturer). This leads to more predictable absorption and fewer amphetamine derivative metabolites. Potentially, this may produce a better adverse event profile than the standard preparation. As a result of the improved

absorption, the dose of the Zelapar formulation is 1.25 or 2.5 mg/d compared with 10 mg/d for the standard product. Data on its long-term efficacy and safety are currently unavailable.

Other potential neuroprotective strategies

Several other drugs have potential neuroprotective properties – these are listed in Table 6.3 and are briefly mentioned below.

- *MAO inhibitors* – new agents are in the process of development (eg rasagiline, lazabemide) but no data on the neuroprotective properties of these drugs are available.

- *Dopamine agonists* – several are currently being evaluated for neuroprotective properties. It is hoped that by reducing potentially damaging overactivity in dopaminergic neurones in PD, agonists may prove to be protective. Studies with ropinirole and low-dose pergolide are eagerly awaited.

Table 6.3
Potential neuroprotective agents in PD

MAO inhibitors	• Selegiline • Rasagiline • Lazabemide
Dopamine agonists	
Growth factors	• Glial-derived nerve growth factor • Brain-derived nerve growth factor
Excitatory amino acid (glutamate) antagonists	• Remacemide
Antioxidants	• Ascorbic acid (vitamin C) • β-carotene • Iron chelators

- *Growth factors* – some, such as glial-derived nerve growth factor, do not cross the blood—brain barrier and must, therefore, be administered directly into the brain either by intraventricular infusion or within viral vectors. These techniques remain experimental.

- *Glutamate antagonists* – the overactivity of the subthalamopallidal glutamatergic pathway in PD has led to the hypothesis that this may, in some way, be neurotoxic. Inhibiting glutamate transmission with remacemide or riluzole may prove neuroprotective and clinical trials are just starting in this area.

- *Antioxidants* – oxidative stress has been invoked as one potential cause of dopaminergic cell death. Antioxidant therapy with the free radical scavenger a-tocopherol (vitamin E) in the DATATOP study failed to be effective. Other potential antioxidants include ascorbic acid (vitamin C), β-carotene, iron chelators and antioxidant enzymes but little or no evidence from clinical trials with these agents is available.

Many other agents, eg growth factors and antioxidants, are being examined for neuroprotective properties

Further reading

Ben-Shlomo Y, Churchyard A, Head J *et al*. Investigation by Parkinson's Disease Research Group of United Kingdom into excess mortality seen with combined levodopa and selegiline treatment in patients with early, mild Parkinson's disease: further results of randomised trial and confidential inquiry. *BMJ* 1998; **316**: 1191–6.

Birkmayer W, Knoll J, Riederer P *et al*. Increased life expectancy resulting from addition of L-deprenyl to madopar treatment in Parkinson's disease: a long-term study. *J Neural Transm* 1985; **64**: 113–27.

Churchyard A, Mathias CJ, Boonkongchuen P, Lees AJ. Autonomic effects of selegiline: possible cardiovascular toxicity in Parkinson's disease. *J Neurol Neurosurg Psychiatry* 1997; **63**: 228–34.

Larsen J, Boas J, Erdal J, The Norwegian-Danish Study Group. Does selegiline modify the progression of early Parkinson's disease? Results from a five-year study. *Eur J Neurol* 1999; **6**: 539–47.

Lees AJ, Parkinson's Disease Research Group of the United Kingdom. Comparison of the therapeutic effects and mortality data of levodopa and levodopa combined with selegiline in patients with early, mild Parkinson's disease. *BMJ* 1995; **311**: 1602–7.

Olanow CW, Hauser RA, Gauger L *et al*. The effect of deprenyl and levodopa on the progression of Parkinson's disease. *Ann Neurol* 1995; **38**: 771–7.

Olanow CW, Myllyla VV, Sotaniemi KA *et al*. Effect of selegiline on mortality in patients with Parkinson's disease. *Neurology* 1998; **51**: 825–30.

The Parkinson Study Group. Mortality in DATATOP: a multicentre trial in early Parkinson's disease. *Ann Neurol* 1998; **43**: 318–25.

The Parkinson Study Group. Impact of deprenyl and tocopherol treatment on Parkinson's disease in DATATOP subjects not receiving levodopa. *Ann Neurol* 1996; **39**: 29–36.

The Parkinson Study Group. Impact of deprenyl and tocopherol treatment on Parkinson's disease in DATATOP patients receiving levodopa. *Ann Neurol* 1996; **39**: 37–45.

The Parkinson Study Group. Effects of tocopherol and deprenyl on the progression of disability in early Parkinson's disease. *N Engl J Med* 1993; **328**: 176–83.

The Parkinson Study Group. Effect of deprenyl on the progression of disability in early Parkinson's disease. *N Engl J Med* 1989; **321**: 1364–71.

Parkinson's Disease Research Group. Comparisons of therapeutic effects of levodopa, levodopa and selegiline, and bromocriptine in patients with early, mild Parkinson's disease: three year interim report. *BMJ* 1993; **307**: 469–72.

Tetrud JW, Langston JW. The effect of deprenyl (selegiline) on the natural history of Parkinson's disease. *Science* 1989; **245**: 519–22.

Thorogood M, Armstrong B, Nichols T, Hollowell J. Mortality in people taking selegiline: observational study. *BMJ* 1998; **317:** 252–4.

Turkka J, Suominen K, Tolonen U *et al.* Selegiline diminishes cardiovascular autonomic responses in Parkinson's disease. *Neurology* 1997; **48:** 662–7.

7. Medical management – symptomatic therapy I: levodopa

Brief history
Pharmacokinetics
Available preparations
Clinical use of immediate-release
    preparations
Associated side-effects
Clinical use of modified-release
    preparations

Brief history

The levodopa story began in 1957 when Carlsson and colleagues demonstrated reversal of akinesia in reserpinized animals following administration of D,L-dopa, suggesting a role for dopamine deficiency in idiopathic Parkinson's disease (PD). Three years later, Ehringer and Hornykiewicz reported dopamine deficiency in the striatum in PD. In 1961, they found, along with Barbeau, that levodopa treatment had a beneficial effect on motor function in PD in small studies. Dopamine itself does not cross the blood–brain barrier. However, these studies used relatively small doses of levodopa which produced such little benefit that its therapeutic potential was nearly missed. Too much levodopa was being metabolized in the periphery and so the amount delivered to the brain was small. It took until 1967 for Cotzias and colleagues to demonstrate dramatic improvement in motor impairments in PD using larger doses of D,L-dopa in just 17 patients.

The therapeutic potential of levodopa was

restricted in these early days by the marked nausea and vomiting associated with it. The development of two peripheral dopa decarboxylase inhibitors – benserazide and carbidopa – in the mid-1970s allowed a reduction in the dose of levodopa while still allowing large amounts to cross the blood–brain barrier. The development of these dopa decarboxylase inhibitors greatly increased the acceptance of levodopa therapy and reduced the cost. However, prescription rates were slow to increase and it took until the late 1980s for these to plateau in the UK, suggesting that all suitable patients were by then receiving levodopa treatment (Figure 7.1).

Pharmacokinetics

Levodopa (Figure 7.2) is absorbed from the small bowel using the large amino acid transport system and is then rapidly distributed with a plasma half-life of 60 minutes; it uses the same active transport mechanism to cross the blood–brain barrier. Consequently, gastric emptying and competition from protein in the diet can interfere with absorption and transfer into the brain. Levodopa is metabolized peripherally and centrally by dopa decarboxylase and catechol-O-methyltransferase (COMT) to dopamine and 3-O-methyldopa respectively (Figure 7.3).

To reduce the peripheral metabolism of levodopa, it is usually administered with a dopa decarboxylase inhibitor such as carbidopa (Sinemet or co-careldopa) or benserazide (Madopar or co-beneldopa). Further peripheral metabolism can be reduced by COMT inhibitors (page 64), such as entacapone and tolcapone, and monoamine oxidase (MAO) B inhibitors (page 35). The pharmacokinetic characteristics of the two modified-release levodopa preparations available are discussed later in this chapter.

Available preparations

As a result of the various combinations of agents and their different doses, many different levodopa preparations are available. This is

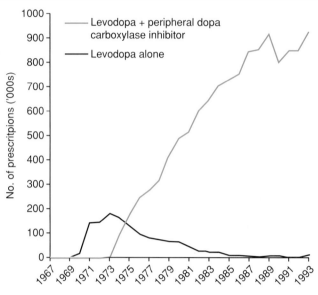

Figure 7.1
Levodopa prescription rates in the UK. Reproduced with permission from IMS Health (Medical Data Index)

confused further by the varied nomenclature used in different countries. Table 7.1 lists the preparations available in the UK.

Clinical use of immediate-release preparations

Levodopa remains the 'gold standard' treatment for PD. Its efficacy is still superior to that of all other available treatments, while its adverse event profile is acceptable. Thus, many patients are still given levodopa once they have significant functional disability. This emphasizes the recommendation that any therapy is held in reserve until the patient has sufficient motor disability to be interfering with

his or her lifestyle. This will vary from patient to patient but it is surprising how well clinicians agree when this point arrives for the individual. For example, the factory worker assembling small components manually will require treatment sooner than will a colleague who uses a computer all day.

> Levodopa remains the 'gold standard' therapy for PD

It is customary to begin with the smallest dose of immediate-release levodopa (with a decarboxylase inhibitor), which will control the patient's symptoms. Many patients can tolerate therapeutic doses immediately, such as Sinemet or Madopar 125 tid with their main meal. However, it is usually best to start older or frail patients on lower doses (eg Sinemet or Madopar 62.5 tid) which are titrated up gradually towards a therapeutic dose over several weeks. All patients will need to be reviewed after one to two months of treatment to assess their response and any side-effects. At this stage, a further increase or even a

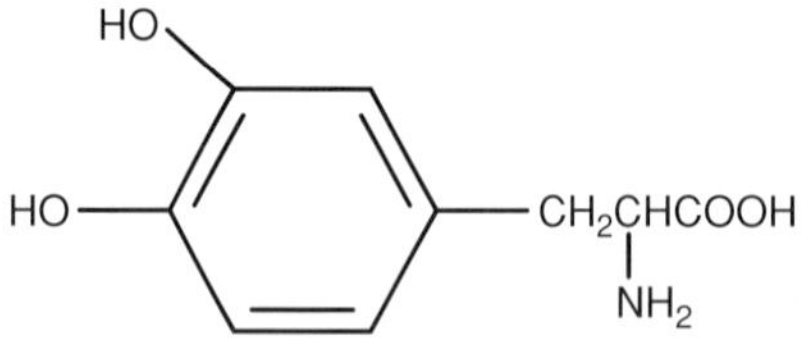

Figure 7.2
Chemical structure of levodopa

Table 7.1
Levodopa preparations available in the UK

Brand name	Generic name	Release mechanism	Levodopa dose (mg)	Decarboxylase dose (mg)
Sinemet LS (low strength)/ Sinemet 62.5	Co-careldopa	Immediate	50	12.5
Sinemet 110	Co-careldopa	Immediate	100	10
Sinemet Plus	Co-careldopa	Immediate	100	25
Sinemet 275	Co-careldopa	Immediate	250	25
Half Sinemet CR	Co-careldopa	Modified-release	100	25
Sinemet CR	Co-careldopa	Modified-release	200	50
Madopar dispersible 62.5	Co-beneldopa	Rapid-release	50	12.5
Madopar dispersible 125	Co-beneldopa	Rapid-release	100	25
Madopar 62.5	Co-beneldopa	Immediate	50	12.5
Madopar 125	Co-beneldopa	Immediate	100	25
Madopar 250	Co-beneldopa	Immediate	200	50
Madopar CR	Co-beneldopa	Modified-release	100	25

decrease in dose may be necessary. Once stabilized in this way, patients are likely to be receiving Sinemet or Madopar 62.5 tid to Sinemet 275 tid/Madopar 250 tid, all doses taken with main meals. Some clinicians presage the need to fractionate immediate-release levodopa doses in later disease by titrating up to Sinemet or Madopar 125 taken five times daily, ie with main meals and 'mid-morning coffee' and 'mid-afternoon tea'.

A number of studies in the late 1970s compared the two immediate-release levodopa preparations available. Although these trials were small and only medium-term (three to six months), no significant differences in efficacy or adverse events were found between Sinemet and Madopar.

Associated side-effects
Short-term effects

Many patients suffer acute side-effects when starting levodopa therapy (Table 7.2). The most common are nausea, loss of appetite and vomiting. Tolerance often develops after several weeks of treatment with complete resolution of symptoms. However, some patients will require treatment with the only available antiemetic which does not cross the blood–brain barrier, domperidone (Motilium) 10–30 mg tid. Postural

hypotension can also occur, but usually settles without the need for treatment. If it does not then an alternative diagnosis should be considered, commonly multiple system atrophy (MSA) (page 23). Sleep disorders triggered by dopaminergic therapy have received little attention in the past, but this is set to change after recent concerns about such disorders with

Table 7.2
Short-term side-effects of levodopa and most other dopaminergic agents

Gastrointestinal:
- Nausea
- Vomiting
- Loss of appetite

Cardiovascular:
- Postural hypotension

Sleep disorder:
- Somnolence
- Insomnia
- Vivid dreams
- Nightmares
- Inversion of sleep–wake cycle

Psychiatric:
- Confusion
- Visual hallucinations
- Delusions
- Illusions

dopamine agonists. Levodopa can cause insomnia, vivid dreams, nightmares, somnolence and an inversion of the sleep–wake cycle. Most of these will resolve with good sleep hygiene and by ensuring the last dose of levodopa is taken in the early evening. Although psychotic adverse events are more commonly seen in late PD, infrequently illusions, visual hallucinations, confusion and delusions occur with early levodopa treatment. This is more likely if the patient is dementing or with combinations of antiparkinsonian drugs.

> Gastrointestinal complications are the most commonly occurring short-term side-effects with levodopa therapy

Long-term complications

As PD progresses, increases in levodopa therapy become necessary and, eventually, patients develop psychiatric and motor side-effects (Table 7.3).

Psychiatric side-effects

Long-term psychiatric effects consist of illusions, visual hallucinations, confusion and delusions. They are often a sign of incipient dementia and otherwise respond to a reduction in the patient's medication load (page 71).

Table 7.3
Long-term complications of levodopa therapy

Involuntary movements:
- Peak-dose choreoathetoid dyskinesia
- Diphasic dyskinesia (at end-of-dose)
- Dystonia (painful cramp in foot)

Response fluctuations:
- End-of-dose deterioration
- Unpredictable 'on'/'off' switching

Psychiatric:
- Confusion
- Visual hallucinations
- Delusions
- Illusions

Motor complications

Motor complications consist of:

- *abnormal involuntary movements (AIMs) or dyskinesias*. The involuntary movements can be athetoid (fluid-twisting movements of the limbs, trunk or face) or choreiform (briefer, jerky, twitching movements, mostly in the limbs). These are usually a peak-dose phenomenon but rarely can recur when the effect of an individual dose wanes, giving rise to a dyskinesia-intermittent-dyskinesia (D-I-D) response, otherwise known as diphasic dyskinesia.

  The other common AIM is dystonia, in which painful muscle contractions cause unusual postures. This can affect the leg, leading to painful plantar flexion and inversion at the ankle and extension of the great toe (so-called 'striatal toe'). Rarely, it can affect the hand. These phenomena frequently occur in the early morning. Dystonia occurred in the days before levodopa therapy and, thus, can be part of the underlying disease process. The increase in dystonia with levodopa therapy clearly links the two but, paradoxically, dystonia often responds to taking a dose of levodopa for reasons which are not understood.

- *response fluctuations*. These include a shortening of the response to each dose of levodopa (end-of-dose deterioration or the wearing off effect) and unpredictable switching between the mobile 'on' phase and the relatively immobile 'off' phase. The latter can occur so rapidly that it resembles the switching on and off of a light switch, a point not often understood by carers and staff.

Motor complications develop in about 50% of all PD patients after six years of therapy, and in 100% of young onset (<40 years) patients after six years of treatment. Similarly, MPTP-treated primates, a more severe model of PD, develop dose-dependent motor complications within days or weeks of first receiving levodopa therapy. In comparison, monotherapy with dopamine agonists (page 53) from the outset in PD does not seem to cause these side-effects. In recent years, it has been concluded that these observations irrevocably link levodopa with such motor complications and, for this reason, levodopa should be held in reserve for as long as possible, if necessary by using other agents in its place. This policy mainly applies to younger patients who will live long enough to develop such complications.

> Long-term use of levodopa causes motor complications that are irreversible, short of neurosurgical intervention

Another argument that is often used to justify delaying levodopa is that it may be toxic. Tissue culture experiments have shown that dopamine and levodopa are both toxic to dopaminergic cells but this has yet to be demonstrated in vivo and in the presence of glial cells. Small postmortem studies of patients without PD who had mistakenly received levodopa for long periods have shown normal dopaminergic cell counts – the levodopa had not damaged their normal dopamine-containing neurones. An unequivocal solution to this argument requires a large study in untreated *de novo* patients, which has just been started by the Parkinson Study Group in North America and is funded by the National Institutes of Health (ELLDOPA Trial).

> Levodopa should be avoided as initial treatment for as long as possible because of its long-term side-effects

The management of motor complications is complex and requires considerable experience in the field. The most simple approach is to fractionate the dose of levodopa. For example, a patient developing complications when receiving Sinemet 275 tid may respond better to Sinemet Plus (125) taken five or six times daily. This reduces the peak effect of levodopa and thus dyskinesia while filling in the gaps between the tid regimen so that end-of-dose deterioration is reduced. However, this can lead

to a sub-threshold dose of levodopa being given so that the patient never switches on. Other approaches involving the addition of dopamine agonist or COMT inhibitor therapy will be discussed in subsequent chapters. Another approach has been to use modified-release preparations of levodopa.

Clinical use of modified-release preparations

Slow- or modified-release preparations of levodopa – Madopar CR and Sinemet CR – were originally developed in an effort to overcome the motor fluctuations seen with long-term therapy in later PD.

Madopar CR

Madopar CR was introduced in the UK in 1988. It was originally labelled Madopar HBS (hydrodynamically balanced system) after its novel release mechanism. When the capsule meets gastric fluid, the gelatine shell undergoes dissolution and a mucous body is formed which floats on the surface of the stomach. It remains in the stomach for prolonged periods of time, releasing levodopa and benserazide through a hydrated layer by diffusion. Pharmacokinetic studies in healthy volunteers and Parkinsonian patients showed that the drug is released and absorbed over a period of four to five hours, maintaining substantial plasma concentrations for six to eight hours after dosing. However, its bioavailability after oral dosing was reduced to 60–70% of that of standard Madopar – this was due to incomplete absorption rather than altered disposition. The presence or absence of food in the stomach had no effect on the absorption of levodopa from Madopar CR.

Sinemet CR

Sinemet CR was introduced in the UK in 1991. It differs from its counterpart in being a slowly eroding, polymer-based matrix containing levodopa and carbidopa. Both are absorbed from the small intestine over four to six hours after oral ingestion. In elderly subjects, the bioavailability of levodopa is reduced in the

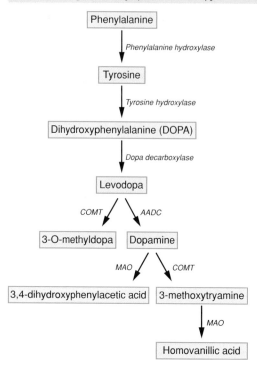

Figure 7.3
Catecholamine biosynthesis and metabolism

Sinemet CR preparation to 70% of that of the standard Sinemet. The bioavailability of levodopa is increased in the presence of food.

Clinical trial results

Clinical trials involving patients with motor complications revealed that both modified-release preparations produced a moderate reduction in 'off' time. The effect on dyskinesia was less predictable although, in general, there tended to be a slight increase. Larger doses of the modified-release preparations were required to achieve this effect. The precise increment varied between studies but an additional 20–60% was necessary. In clinical trials, both clinicians and patients preferred the modified-release formulation to the immediate-release preparation. The adverse event profile was similar for standard and modified-release agents. There was also a reduction in the number of daily doses of modified-release

levodopa compared with the standard formulation in patients with later disease from an average of five to between three and four doses per day. Advice on conversion from an immediate- to modified-release preparation is provided in Table 7.4. A study of healthy volunteers showed that the pharmacological profile of the two preparations was equivalent, and the small comparative studies suggest they produce similar clinical benefits.

Two studies have examined the use of modified-release levodopa in early untreated disease in the hope of preventing long-term motor complications. The first of these was a randomized double-blind parallel-group multicentre study of 134 Danish-Norwegian patients with untreated *de novo* PD randomized to receive Madopar CR or standard Madopar. After five years, there was no significant difference in the frequency of motor fluctuations (57% v 59% for Madopar CR and standard Madopar respectively) or dyskinesia (34% v 41% for Madopar CR and standard Madopar respectively). The analogous study with Sinemet CR was also well conducted in a randomized triple-blind (ie statistical analysis was also performed blind) parallel-group design

Table 7.4
Advice on conversion of a patient with motor complications from immediate- to modified-release levodopa

- Convert patient to CR preparation overnight
- Give 40–50% more CR preparation than previous immediate-release
- Increase intervals between CR doses (eg start with three main meals)
- Add a small dose of immediate-release (eg 62.5–125) with breakfast as a 'kick-start'
- See the patient after one to two weeks to adjust doses or ask the PD nurse specialist (chapter 12) to do this
- Adjust dose and timing of CR and add more immediate-release doses with meals as necessary
- For increased latency to effect, consider increasing immediate-release, CR or both
- For build-up of dyskinesia or psychosis later in the day, reduce CR and increase immediate-release

in 35 centres worldwide. A total of 618 untreated patients were randomized in what was called the CR First Study. After five years, there was no significant difference in motor fluctuations between those receiving standard Sinemet and those on Sinemet CR (16% in both groups). The low incidence of fluctuations compared with other studies was due to the strict criteria used to define the presence of fluctuations in this trial. Interestingly, a small and statistically significant advantage of Sinemet CR in terms of the Unified Parkinson's Disease Rating Scale (UPDRS) activity in daily life (ADL) score was found at five years. These trials concluded that the present modified-release levodopa preparations are no better than standard levodopa with regard to the genesis of motor complications. There is, therefore, no justification for using these more expensive agents in *de novo* PD.

One particularly valuable place for modified-release levodopa is in patients with nocturnal hypokinesia. This can significantly improve mobility throughout the night, allowing patients to turn in bed more freely and to reach the toilet without the assistance of a carer. There can also be beneficial effects left by the following morning so that the patient has a longer period of sleep benefit. Large doses must be avoided as these can produce nightmares, confusion and/or hallucinations.

> Modified-release levodopa preparations are particularly useful for nocturnal hypokinesia

Further reading

Block G, Liss C, Reines S *et al*. Comparison of immediate-release and controlled-release carbidopa/levodopa in Parkinson's disease. *Eur Neurol* 1997; **37:** 23–7.

Clarke CE. Modified-release drugs for Parkinson's disease. *Prescriber* 1997; **8:** 85–90.

Clarke CE, Sambrook MA, Mitchell IJ, Crossman AR. Levodopa-induced dyskinesia and response fluctuations in primates rendered parkinsonian with 1-methyl-4-phenyl-1,2,3,6-tetrahydropyridine (MPTP). *J Neurol Sci* 1987; **78:** 273–80.

Clarke CE, Sampaio C. Movement Disorders Cochrane Collaborative Review Group. *Mov Disord* 1997; **12:** 477–82.

Cotzias GC, Woert MHV, Schiffer LM. Aromatic amino acids and modification of parkinsonism. *N Engl J Med* 1967; **276:** 374–9.

Diamond SG, Markham CH, Treciokas LJ. A double-blind comparison of levodopa, Madopa, and Sinemet in Parkinson's disease. *Ann Neurol* 1978; **3:** 267–72.

Dupont E, Anderson A, Boas J *et al*. Sustained-release Madopar HBS compared with standard Madopar in the long-term treatment of de novo parkinsonian patients. *Acta Neurol Scand* 1996; **93:** 14–20.

Fahn S. Parkinson disease, the effect of levodopa, and the ELLDOPA trial. Earlier vs Later L-DOPA. *Arch Neurol* 1999; **56:** 529–35.

Fahn S. Welcome news about levodopa, but uncertainty remains. *Ann Neurol* 1998; **43:** 550–3.

Markham CH, Diamond SG, Treciokas LJ. Carbidopa in Parkinson's disease and in nausea and vomiting of levodopa. *Arch Neurol* 1974; **31:** 128–33.

Pakkenberg H, Birket-Smith E, Dupont E *et al*. Parkinson's disease treated with Sinemet or Madopar: a controlled multicentre study. *Acta Neurol Scand* 1976; **3:** 76–85.

Poewe W, Granata R. Pharmacological treatment of Parkinson's disease. In: Watts RL, Koller WC, eds. *Movement disorders: neurologic principles and practice*. New York: McGraw-Hill, 1997: 201–9.

Quinn N, Critchley P, Parkes D, Marsden CD. When should levodopa be started? *Lancet* 1986; **2:** 985–6.

Rajput AH, Stern W, Laverty WH. Chronic low-dose levodopa therapy in Parkinson's disease: an argument for delaying levodopa therapy. *Neurology* 1984; **34:** 991–6.

Rajput AJ, Fenton ME, Birdi S, Macaulay R. Is levodopa toxic to human substantia nigra? *Mov Disord* 1997; **12:** 634–8.

Rinne UK, Molsa P. Levodopa with benserazide or carbidopa in Parkinson's disease. *Neurology* 1979; **29:** 1584–9.

8. Medical management – symptomatic therapy II: dopamine agonists

Brief history
Pharmacokinetics
Adverse effects and prevention
Monotherapy
Adjuvant therapy
Apomorphine

motor complications. Later studies with older agonists raised the possibility that dopamine agonist monotherapy in the early stages of the disease produces fewer motor complications than levodopa. More recently, this led to large, long-term monotherapy trials with the newer agonists, such as ropinirole, pergolide, cabergoline and pramipexole, the results of which will be discussed in this chapter.

Pharmacokinetics

Six oral dopamine agonists are licensed in the UK and one agent that is administered parenterally, apomorphine. There are two groups of dopamine receptor: the D_1 and the D_2 receptor 'families' (Figure 8.1).

Table 8.1 summarizes the basic pharmacology of the dopamine agonists. The oral agents will

Brief history

The first oral dopamine agonists entered clinical practice in the late 1970s. Agonists act directly on postsynaptic dopamine receptors in the striatum without the need for conversion to dopamine, unlike levodopa (chapter 7). They, therefore, bypass the degenerating nigrostriatal dopaminergic neurones and so it was hoped that they would prove more effective than levodopa in the later stages of idiopathic Parkinson's Disease (PD), and perhaps be better tolerated. Correspondingly, the initial work with the older agonists such as bromocriptine was as adjuvant or add-on therapy in patients with

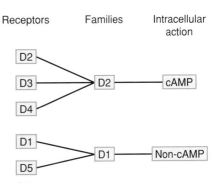

Figure 8.1
Dopamine receptor subtypes. cAMP = cyclic adenosine monophosphate

Table 8.1
Pharmacology of the dopamine agonists

Agonist	D_2 group affinity	D_1 group affinity	Ergot-derived	Half-life (h)	T_{max}	Clearance
Bromocriptine	+++	–	Yes	3–6	1.2 h	Hepatic metabolism
Lisuride	++	0/–	Yes	2–3	1 h	Hepatic metabolism
Pergolide	+++	+	Yes	15–42	2 h	Renal excretion
Ropinirole	+++	0	No	3–5	1–2 h	Hepatic metabolism
Cabergoline	+++	0	Yes	65	0.5–4.0 h	Hepatic metabolism
Pramipexole	+++	0	No	8–12	1–3 h	Renal excretion (90%)
Apomorphine	+++	+++	No	0.5	8 min	Hepatic metabolism

+ = agonist; – = antagonist; 0/– = partial antagonist

be considered separately from apomorphine, which is discussed at the end of the chapter.

Adverse effects and prevention

The side-effect profiles of the dopamine agonists are similar to those of levodopa but such problems occur more frequently and/or with greater severity. The most commonly experienced are:

- nausea
- vomiting
- reduced appetite
- postural hypotension
- confusion
- hallucinations
- somnolence.

> The side-effects associated with dopamine agonists are similar to those of levodopa but occur more frequently

Most of these can be avoided by slow titration of the agonist, which is usually supervised by the patient's general practitioner. Tables 8.2–8.6 provide details of the titration regimens of the commonly used agonists which should be of value in clinical practice.

Starter packs of pergolide and ropinirole are available to make titration easier for the patient. Gastrointestinal problems can be blocked with the peripheral dopamine D_2 receptor antagonist domperidone (10–20 mg tid). Tolerance to these dopaminergic effects

Table 8.2
Bromocriptine titration regimen (initial therapeutic range: monotherapy and adjuvant therapy 10–40 mg/d)

Week 1	1–1.25 mg at night
Week 2	2–2.5 mg at night
Week 3	2.5 mg bd
Week 4	2.5 mg tid
Then every 3–10 days	Add 2.5 mg/day

Table 8.3
Pergolide titration regimen (initial therapeutic range: monotherapy and adjuvant therapy 1.5–3.0 mg/d)

Days 1 and 2	50 µg once at night
Days 3 and 4	50 µg tid
Days 5 and 6	50 + 100 + 100 µg daily
Days 7 and 8	100 + 100 + 150 µg daily
Days 9 and 10	150 µg tid
Days 11 and 12	200 µg tid
Days 13 and 14	250 µg tid
Then every three days	Add 250 µg/day

Table 8.4
Ropinirole titration regimen (initial therapeutic range: monotherapy 8–12 mg/d; adjuvant therapy 12–24 mg/d)

Week 1	0.25 mg tid
Week 2	0.5 mg tid
Week 3	0.75 mg tid
Week 4	1 mg tid
Week 5	2 + 1 + 1 mg daily
Week 6	2 + 2 + 1 mg daily
Week 7	2 mg tid
Week 8	4 + 2 + 2 mg daily
Week 9	4 + 4 + 2 mg daily
Week 10	4 mg tid
Week 11	5 mg tid
Week 12	6 mg tid
Week 13	7 mg tid
Week 14	8 mg tid

Table 8.5
Cabergoline titration regimen (initial therapeutic range 2–4 mg/d)

Week 1	1 mg once daily
Week 2	2 mg once daily
Week 3	3 mg once daily
Week 4	4 mg once daily
Week 5	5 mg once daily
Week 6	6 mg once daily

also develops over several weeks of treatment. Ergot-derived agonists can also cause their own specific problems such as ankle oedema, erythromelalgia (ie florid erythema and swelling, usually of the lower limb), Raynaud's phenomenon, and serosal complications such as retroperitoneal fibrosis and pleural effusion.

Table 8.6
Pramipexole titration regimen – as hydrochloride salt
(initial therapeutic range 1.5–3.0 mg/d)

Week 1	0.125 mg tid
Week 2	0.25 mg tid
Week 3	0.5 mg tid
Week 4	0.75 mg tid
Week 5	1 mg tid
Week 6	1.25 mg tid
Week 7	1.5 mg tid

Monotherapy

After the value of dopamine agonists was demonstrated in adjuvant therapy trials, research turned to assessing their ability in early PD to prevent motor complications by acting as:

- sole therapy without any levodopa (monotherapy)
- levodopa-sparing agents in combination therapy with levodopa.

After several trials with bromocriptine and one with lisuride, long-term monotherapy trials of the latest dopamine agonists were set up which have only recently been reported. These trials have had a fundamental impact on the way PD is treated, at least in 'younger' patients.

> Dopamine agonists may be used as an alternative to levodopa as monotherapy

Bromocriptine trials

Two systematic reviews under the auspices of the Cochrane Movement Disorders Collaborative Review Group have evaluated bromocriptine in patients with early PD as:

- *pure monotherapy versus levodopa on its own* – this found only six randomized control trials (RCTs) with follow-up for one-and-a-half to five years in about 850 patients. There was significantly less dyskinesia in one of the three studies in which this was measured. There was no

significant reduction in motor fluctuations and motor impairment, and disability rating scales were too diverse to reach any conclusions. However, adverse events were worse in the bromocriptine arms of these studies. It was concluded that bromocriptine monotherapy could delay the onset of dyskinesia in those who were able to tolerate it

- *combination therapy with levodopa versus levodopa alone* – this found a further six RCTs with follow-up for one-and-a-half to five years in 898 patients. There was only a trend for less dyskinesia in the combination therapy group with no difference in fluctuations. Again, impairment and disability scales were too diverse to interpret and there were significantly more adverse events in the bromocriptine/ levodopa arms of the trials. It was concluded that there was no advantage in combination therapy with bromocriptine from the outset.

> Levodopa should be avoided as initial therapy at least in younger patients to avoid long-term complications such as dyskinesia and on/off fluctuations

Lisuride trial

Only one RCT has examined the effect of lisuride therapy in early PD. In this trial, 90 patients were randomized to receive lisuride, lisuride/levodopa or levodopa over a four-year period. Most patients taking only lisuride added levodopa at a later stage as 'rescue' medication when the effects of lisuride were insufficient, even after dose titration. This prevented a firm conclusion about lisuride monotherapy. The lisuride/levodopa combination group, however, showed significantly less dyskinesia and motor fluctuations than the pure levodopa group. Efficacy in terms of motor impairments and disability was not different between the groups at the end of four years. The authors suggested that combination therapy with an agonist such as lisuride and levodopa should be the first-line choice in early PD.

> Data on bromocriptine and lisuride monotherapy are insufficient to support their use as monotherapy

Ropinirole trial

The results of dopamine agonist monotherapy trials thus far were generally thought to be equivocal and it was decided that more conclusive data were needed before a fundamental move away from levodopa therapy in early disease was made. It was the trial of ropinirole monotherapy that provided this conclusive data and led to a change in practice. This double-blind controlled trial randomized 268 patients with early PD to:

* *ropinirole monotherapy* – to which levodopa could be added later as 'rescue' treatment (n=179)
* *levodopa alone*, with potential levodopa rescue (n=89).

There was a reduced risk of dyskinesia in patients treated with initial ropinirole monotherapy than levodopa monotherapy; after five years, only 20% of those in the ropinirole arm had dyskinesia compared with 45% in the levodopa arm (hazard ratio 3.8; 95% CI 2.1,

6.9; p<0.0001) (Figure 8.2). No difference in motor fluctuations was seen but 'on'/'off' diary cards were not recorded in this early disease study. Some debate has surrounded the analysis method of the activities of daily living (ADL) and motor function scale – parts II and III of the Unified Parkinson's Disease Rating Scale respectively – but any differences were small and only significant at the five-year time point for the motor score in favour of levodopa (Figure 8.3). Adverse events were similar between the two groups, apart from a significant increase in hallucinations with ropinirole. It was concluded that initial monotherapy with ropinirole with the later addition of levodopa could significantly delay the development of dyskinesia, which was a worthy aim, at least in younger patients.

Pergolide trial

Until recently, only bromocriptine, lisuride and ropinirole were licensed for use as monotherapy in PD in the UK. Pergolide has only just been granted a monotherapy product licence; despite this, it has been used as a monotherapy agent for many years. The preliminary report of a three-year double-blind RCT in 294 PD patients was recently released comparing pergolide with levodopa as monotherapy. This study differed from the other recent monotherapy trials in that supplemental levodopa was not allowed in

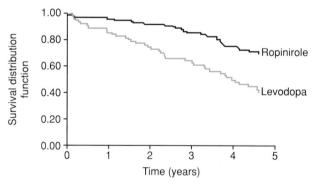

Figure 8.2
Rate of development of dyskinesia in patients with initial ropinirole monotherapy versus levodopa monotherapy.
Reproduced with permission from Rascol O *et al. N Engl J Med* 2000; **342**: 1484–91

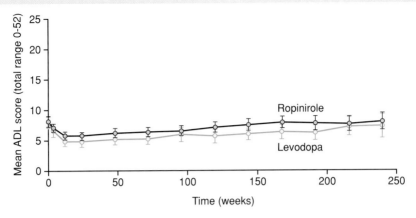

Figure 8.3
UPDRS ADL scores for patients randomized to initial ropinirole monotherapy or levodopa monotherapy. Reproduced with permission from Rascol O *et al. N Engl J Med* 2000; **342**: 1484–91

the agonist arm. The primary endpoint was the time to onset of motor complications, defined as the first positive UPDRS complications of therapy (part IV) rating. After three years, 16% of patients taking pergolide had reached the endpoint compared to 33% in the levodopa group (*p*=0.004). Both the times to onset of dyskinesia and motor fluctuations were significantly delayed with pergolide monotherapy. However, UPDRS motor ratings at the end of three years were worse on pergolide and there were more withdrawals due to adverse events in the pergolide arm (18% v 10%, *p*<0.05).

Cabergoline trial

The preliminary findings of a long-term cabergoline monotherapy trial have recently been reported. In this double-blind RCT, 419 patients were randomized to:

- initial cabergoline monotherapy with later levodopa 'rescue' if necessary (*n*=211)
- levodopa with potential levodopa 'rescue' (*n*=208).

After five years, 22% of the cabergoline group had motor complications compared with 34% of the levodopa group (*p*<0.05). The relatively low prevalence of total complications, even in the levodopa group, was probably due to the strict

requirement for the recording of motor complications at two consecutive visits. No further details of the results of this trial are available at present.

Pramipexole trial

In a double-blind RCT examining pramipexole monotherapy, 301 patients were randomized to:

- initial pramipexole monotherapy with the potential for levodopa 'rescue' as required
- levodopa with possible levodopa rescue.

After mean follow-up of 23.5 months, 28% in the pramipexole group had one or more motor complications compared with 51% in the levodopa group (hazard ratio 0.44; 95% CI 0.30, 0.66; *p*<0.0001). There was a significant reduction in dyskinesia, in the wearing-off phenomenon, and in unpredictable 'on'-'off' fluctuations in the pramipexole arm. However, those on pramipexole had significantly less improvement in UPDRS motor scores despite availability of rescue levodopa therapy.

Summary

It appears that all oral dopamine agonists used as initial monotherapy (with the later addition of levodopa when necessary) can delay the development of dyskinesia and probably motor fluctuations in early PD. These findings have led to 'younger' patients who will live long enough to develop motor complications being given agonist monotherapy.

> Recently published trials with cabergoline, pergolide, pramipexole, and ropinirole monotherapy show that these agents can delay the onset of motor complications

However, this fundamental change in treatment policy does not take into account the additional cost of agonists compared with the relatively inexpensive levodopa. No health economics assessments were performed in any of the recently reported trials. Admittedly, dyskinesia is irreversible once it has developed, with the exception of expensive surgical intervention. So, it is possible that by delaying the onset of dyskinesia, fewer patients will require surgery and thus, in the long-term (at least 10 years), costs will be reduced. Healthcare systems need rapidly to address this issue. The PD MED Trial, recently begun by the University of Birmingham Clinical Trials Unit, will focus on this problem. In the early disease randomization, between 1,500 and 3,000 PD patients will be randomized to any levodopa preparation, dopamine agonist and MAO B inhibitor, although the clinician can opt out from the MAO B inhibitor or the levodopa arms in individual cases. In addition to following quality of life (PDQ 39 and EuroQol, page 69) and mortality for at least 10 years, there will be regular health economics assessments. This will allow a class effect comparison between agonists and levodopa in terms of quality of life and healthcare costs. As a pragmatic 'real-life' trial which is likely to randomize patients older than those who usually enter PD trials, it will also provide information on the use of agonist monotherapy in older patients. At present we have no useful data on which age groups should be given such treatment.

> Further work is needed to assess the impact of agonist monotherapy on quality of life and health economics across the full age spectrum of PD patients

Adjuvant therapy

The initial trials with oral dopamine agonist therapy were carried out in patients on levodopa who had developed motor complications. The aims of such adjuvant treatment are to:

- reduce the amount of time the patient spends in the relatively immobile 'off' phase
- reduce the dose of levodopa in the hope of minimizing motor complications in the future
- improve motor impairments, disability and handicap.

These aims should be achieved with an acceptable increase in dyskinesia (which is inevitable with any increase in treatment at this stage in the condition) and other adverse events.

Fortunately, the plethora of RCTs in this area have recently undergone systematic review through the Cochrane Movement Disorders Collaborative Review Group. As a result, a valuable synthesis of the data on all agonists available in the UK is now available electronically on the Cochrane Library. The Cochrane review of placebo-controlled trials of adjuvant bromocriptine therapy in PD reported such heterogeneity in trial design and outcome that no conclusion on its efficacy and safety could be reached. Although lack of evidence of effect does not imply lack of effect, this is intriguing since bromocriptine has been the 'gold standard' agonist with which the modern agonists have all been compared.

The remaining 10 Cochrane adjuvant dopamine agonist therapy reviews reported on 11 RCTs (two unpublished) which compared cabergoline, pergolide, pramipexole and ropinirole with placebo in 1,596 patients. A total of 13 bromocriptine-controlled trials (six unpublished) were found with all of the above agonists in 2,029 patients. No placebo-controlled studies with lisuride were found and the only bromocriptine-controlled study was small and contained little relevant data. The results and implications of these studies are summarized below but further details are available in the individual Cochrane reviews on the Cochrane Library.

Meta-analysis of the placebo-controlled trials showed that 'off' time significantly improved with cabergoline, pergolide and pramipexole. The absence of significant 'off' time reduction with ropinirole was due to imbalance in the severity of parkinsonism between the active and the control arms in the single phase III study. Dyskinesia reported as an adverse event was significantly worse with the modern agonists compared with placebo. The UPDRS motor and ADL scales and their predecessors were not measured in all of these studies. However, significant improvements were noted in both of these scales in most trials with cabergoline and pramipexole. The Columbia scale improved with pergolide in the one RCT where this was measured. Levodopa dose was significantly reduced with all modern agonists.

> For patients already on levodopa who have developed motor complications, adjuvant dopamine agonist therapy can reduce 'off' time, levodopa dose and motor impairments, but at the expense of more dyskinesia

Overview of adverse events in the placebo-controlled trials is hampered by incomplete reporting but meta-analysis showed significantly more nausea, hallucinations and somnolence with the agonists. The latter has recently become a matter of some concern when so-called 'sleep attacks' were reported in a small number of patients taking pramipexole and in one case ropinirole. More recently, it has been shown that daytime somnolence is an issue for up to 75% of patients and that this and the

sudden onset of sleep can occur with all dopaminergic agents. Despite these problems, meta-analysis of all-cause withdrawal rates showed significantly fewer drop-outs with the dopamine agonists.

No clear superiority of one agonist over another emerged from the placebo-controlled trials. Direct head-to-head comparisons would be required to demonstrate this.

Are the modern agonists significantly better than the less expensive bromocriptine as adjuvant therapy? There was a trend with cabergoline, pramipexole and ropinirole for more 'off' time reduction individually which reached statistical significance on meta-analysis of all of the trials. The modern agents produced about 30 minutes less 'off' time daily than bromocriptine. This is around the value most patients and clinicians would feel is worthwhile, but whether or not this is worth the additional cost is uncertain since we do not have sufficient health economics data for the UK population to assess this. No difference between modern agonists and bromocriptine was seen in dyskinesia, levodopa dose reduction or all cause withdrawal rate and no consistent differences in measures of motor impairment and disability were found.

Using the information from these reviews, it is clear that a trial comparing the four modern agonists with bromocriptine would be prohibitively large and of little clinical value unless unexpectedly large changes emerged. Thus, although the recently introduced agonists have some advantage over bromocriptine, a choice between cabergoline, pergolide, pramipexole and ropinirole must be made on the basis of factors other than efficacy and safety; issues such as dose frequency, ease of titration and affordability must be taken into account.

> Insufficient evidence is available on which to base a choice between the modern agonists, but factors such as dose frequency, ease of titration and affordability should be considered

Apomorphine

Brief history

Apomorphine is an extremely potent D_1 and D_2 dopamine agonist which was used for many years as an emetic. Its bioavailability is poor after oral administration because of extensive first pass metabolism in the liver. Large doses were used in early studies such that the induced emesis caused pre-renal failure and the cessation of further trials.

> Apomorphine is a potent dopamine agonist available as a subcutaneous injection or infusion

Its role as a therapy in PD was developed in London in the late 1980s by Drs Andrew Lees and Gerald Stern. This was facilitated by the availability of the antiemetic domperidone which, in doses of 10–30 mg tid, can prevent most gastrointestinal problems caused by apomorphine. Subcutaneous bolus doses or continuous infusions of apomorphine were effective in reversing 'off' periods even in patients with severe fluctuations in response with a latency of 10–15 minutes. This and most of the subsequent studies were non-randomized and uncontrolled, but just recently small placebo controlled studies have confirmed the benefits of intermittent apomorphine injections. No health economics analysis of this costly treatment (about £10,000/patient/year for continuous infusion) has been performed. However, the beneficial effects in the highly selected small population of patients with severe motor fluctuations are such that many other costs are offset by this treatment, most importantly nursing home placement.

> Intermittent injections can reverse 'off' periods for a while until oral medication takes effect. For patients with many 'off' periods per day, continuous apomorphine infusion can be a very effective treatment

Clinical use

Apomorphine therapy is only suitable for use in specialized centres with experience in the technique and usually with a PD nurse specialist (chapter 12).

- The patient is admitted for an acute apomorphine challenge test under domperidone cover, often performed by the nurse.

- In the 'off' phase, the patient is given an initial dose of around 1 mg subcutaneous escalating at 30-minute intervals through 2, 3, 4 and 6 mg if necessary until a response is seen in motor impairments, which is measured by timed tests of motor function (eg tapping 20 times on two spots 30 cm apart).

- Once the threshold dose (usually 2–4 mg) has been established, the patient with five or six 'off' periods per day is given the same number of bolus apomorphine injections just above this dose at the onset of his or her 'off' period.

- If successful in reducing 'off' time, the patient is trained to use a special Penject injection system (Figure 8.4) which simplifies the process by being pre-filled with apomorphine and having a dial which allows the dose to be easily chosen.

> The significant cost of apomorphine infusions is offset by keeping patients out of nursing homes

Subcutaneous infusions of apomorphine are used for patients with so many 'off' periods that repeated single dose injections are inappropriate. The drug is drawn up once or twice daily and placed in a portable syringe driver. This is connected to a butterfly cannula which is sited once daily in the abdominal wall or subcutaneous tissue of the thighs. The pump can be programmed to deliver in the range of 50–120 mg apomorphine over either the waking day or the whole 24-hour period. The patient's oral medication can then be reduced according to his or her response. Many are able to

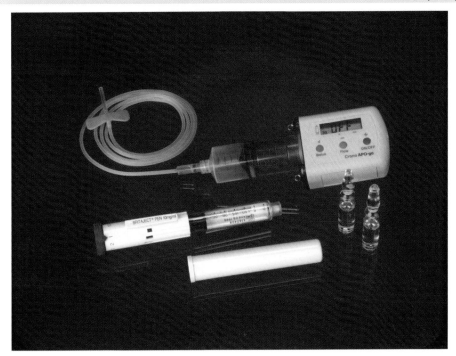

Figure 8.4
Apomorphine infusion pump and Penject injection system

withdraw oral agonists and reduce their levodopa dose substantially. The 'fine tuning' required with this technique is difficult without the benefit of a PD nurse specialist who can visit the patient at home. Continuous infusions are not without hazard. The most common is injection site reactions with the oxidized apomorphine irritating the overlying skin causing large bruises and pain (Figure 8.5). Regular rotation of infusion sites and ultrasonic stimulation can help this problem.

> A PD nurse specialist is crucial in monitoring apomorphine therapy

More recently, the intensive use of continuous 'waking day' apomorphine infusions in patients with severe dyskinesia has shown that it can reduce dyskinesia by 65% in severity and 85% in frequency and duration. This suggests that it

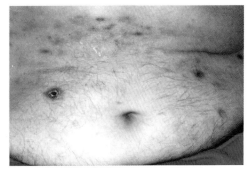

Figure 8.5
Infusion site reactions with apomorphine

is an alternative to invasive surgical procedures in such patients.

The need for the parenteral administration of apomorphine makes it impractical for many patients. Attempts are underway to create more acceptable delivery methods such as sublingual, transdermal and rectal routes, but intranasal administration led to unacceptable local inflammation.

Further reading

Cochrane Collaboration website: http://www.cochrane.org.

Colzi A, Turner K, Lees AJ. Continuous subcutaneous waking day apomorphine in the long-term treatment of levodopa-induced interdose dyskinesias in Parkinson's disease. *J Neurol Neurosurg Psychiatry* 1998; **64:** 573–6.

Cotzias G, Papavasiliou P, Tolosa ES *et al.* Treatment of Parkinson's disease with apomorphine: possible role of growth hormone. *N Engl J Med* 1976; **294:** 567–72.

Ferreira JJ, Desboeuf K, Galitzky M *et al.* 'Sleep attacks' and Parkinson's disease: results of a questionnaire survey in a movement disorders outpatient clinic. *Mov Disord* 2000; **15**(suppl 3): 187.

Frankel JP, Lees AJ, Kempster PA, Stern GM. Subcutaneous apomorphine in the treatment of Parkinson's disease. *J Neurol Neurosurg Psychiatry* 1990; **53:** 96–101.

Frucht S, Rogers JD, Greene PE *et al.* Falling asleep at the wheel: motor vehicle mishaps in persons taking pramipexole and ropinirole. *Neurology* 1999; **52:** 1908–10.

Hutton JT, Dewey RB, LeWitt PA, Factor SA. A randomised double-blind placebo-controlled trial of subcutaneously injected apomorphine for parkinsonian off states. *Mov Disord* 2000; **15**(suppl 3): 130.

Lieberman AN, Goldstein M. Treatment of advanced Parkinson's disease with dopamine agonists. In: Marsden CD, Fahn S, eds. *Movement disorders*. London: Butterworth, 1982: 146–65.

Oertel WH. Pergolide versus levodopa monotherapy (PELMOPET). *Mov Disord* 2000; **15**(suppl 3): 4.

Parkinson Study Group. Pramipexole versus levodopa as initial treatment for Parkinson's disease. *JAMA* 2000; **284:** 1931–8.

Poewe W, Granata R. Pharmacological treatment of Parkinson's disease. In: Watts RL, Koller WC, eds. *Movement disorders: neurologic principles and practice.* New York: McGraw-Hill, 1997: 201–19.

Ramaker C, van Hilten J. Bromocriptine/levodopa versus levodopa in early Parkinson's disease. *Parkinsonism and Related Disorders* 1999; **5**(suppl): 82.

Ramaker C, van Hilten JJ. Bromocriptine versus levodopa in early Parkinson's disease. *Parkinsonism and Related Disorders* 1999; **5**(suppl): 83.

Rascol O, Brooks D, Korczyn A *et al.* Early treatment with ropinirole reduces the risk of dyskinesia in Parkinson's disease: a 5-year randomised levodopa-controlled study. *N Engl J Med* 2000; **342:** 1484–91.

Rinne UK. A 5 year double blind study with cabergoline versus levodopa in the treatment of early Parkinson's disease. *Parkinsonism Relat Disord* 1999; **5**(suppl): S84.

Rinne UK. Lisuride, a dopamine agonist in the treatment of early Parkinson's disease. *Neurology* 1989; **39:** 336–9.

van Hilten JJ, Ramaker C, van de Beek WJT, Finken MJJ. Bromocriptine for levodopa-induced motor complications in Parkinson's disease (Cochrane Review). Oxford: Update Software, 1999.

9. Medical management – symptomatic therapy III: other therapies

Anticholinergic agents
Amantadine
Selegiline
COMT inhibitors
Propranolol

Anticholinergic agents

Brief history

The anticholinergics are the oldest of the pharmacotherapies for idiopathic Parkinson's disease (PD). They first emerged in the late 19th century after Charcot's studies with hyoscine (scopolamine). It was not until the mid-20th century that relatively selective centrally active muscarinic receptor antagonists were developed with fewer peripheral side-effects. In the absence of alternatives, these agents proliferated and a large number are still technically available (Table 9.1). The most commonly used in neurology are benzhexol and orphenadrine.

> Benzhexol and orphenadrine are the most commonly used anticholinergics in the UK for the treatment of PD

Mode of action

The precise pharmacodynamic action of the muscarinic antagonists is not clear. Generations of medical students have been taught that a 'balance' existed between cholinergic overactivity and dopaminergic underactivity in PD. This concept is too simplistic and the precise relationship between the two neurotransmitter pathways remains uncertain.

Clinical use

With the introduction of the more effective levodopa (chapter 7), the use of anticholinergics declined. The recognition in recent years of significant cognitive impairment with these drugs, even in normal volunteers, has led to a further reluctance to use them. They should now be restricted to young PD patients with severe tremor, for whom they may be more effective than levodopa.

> Anticholinergics should only be prescribed to young patients with severe tremor or dystonia

Even in these patients, central side-effects may be dose-limiting. These agents can help severe dystonia but paradoxically may aggravate choreoathetoid dyskinesia. The use of anticholinergics as monotherapy to delay the introduction of levodopa has now largely been supplanted by dopamine agonists (chapter 8). Clinical trials with all the muscarinic antagonists were performed many years ago and do not stand up to modern scrutiny. Thus, most of the current advice on their use is based on

Table 9.1
Anticholinergic agents licensed in the UK for the treatment of PD

Generic name	Brand name	Therapeutic dose range
Benzhexol (US trihexyphenidyl)	Broflex, Artane	2–5 mg tid
Orphenadrine	Biorphen, Disipal	50 mg bd or tid
Procyclidine	Arpicolin, Kemadrin	5–10 mg tid
Benztropine	Cogentin	1–2 mg tid
Biperiden	Akineton	2–4 mg tid

common clinical experience rather than hard evidence.

Adverse effects

The main drawback of this class of drugs is the high adverse event profile. Confusion, hallucinations and cognitive impairment are the main problems associated with the central nervous system. Peripheral side-effects include nausea, dry mouth, constipation, dizziness, blurred vision, precipitation of closed-angle glaucoma, and urinary retention in prostatic hypertrophy. These are more common in the elderly, in whom the anticholinergic agents should be avoided. Caution should be exercised when withdrawing an anticholinergic at any age as it may have been surprisingly efficacious. An increase in the patient's additional antiparkinsonian medication will be required in most cases.

> Anticholinergic use is limited by side-effects including confusion, hallucinations, cognitive impairment and urinary retention

Amantadine
Brief history

The discovery of the therapeutic value of amantadine in PD was purely fortuitous. During studies carried out in patients with viral illnesses, amantadine was given to a patient with PD who showed a significant improvement in motor function. As a result, a series of small randomized placebo-controlled trials were performed with amantadine in the condition in the early 1970s. Following encouraging results, the drug was introduced into clinical practice.

Mode of action

The mechanism of the central action of amantadine in PD is still uncertain. In the past, actions via dopaminergic and/or cholinergic pathways have been suggested. More recently, it has been found to be a glutamate antagonist.

Clinical use

The original clinical trials with amantadine in PD suffered from a number of problems, including:

- their small size
- the variety of unvalidated clinical rating scales used
- the mixture of PD and post-encephalitic cases
- the inclusion of patients who had undergone thalamotomy.

However, these studies did demonstrate a beneficial effect on motor impairments. The controlled trials were predominantly short-term (<12 weeks) but the few long-term controlled and observational studies suggested that tolerance to the effects of amantadine developed with use over 12 weeks. Considering the quality of these trials, such tolerance should be viewed cautiously.

In the past, amantadine was used to delay levodopa therapy in a similar manner to the anticholinergics. This role has now been replaced by the dopamine agonists which may be more effective in treating motor impairments and delaying motor complications, although no direct comparative evidence of this exists. Doses in the range of 100 mg bd or tid can be used with no need for further titration. More recently, amantadine has been examined as an antidyskinetic agent based on the knowledge that it is a glutamate antagonist and that dyskinesia may be mediated through an overactive glutamatergic subthalamopallidal pathway. Early pilot studies have provided encouraging results, but larger and longer trials are now needed before amantadine can be recommended to treat dyskinesia.

> Until larger trials are carried out, amantadine should only be prescribed for patients with moderate to severe dyskinesia

Adverse effects

Adverse events can be a significant problem with amantadine. Central side-effects such as confusion and hallucinations can occur, and peripheral reactions include ankle oedema and livedo reticularis.

> Amantadine use is limited by side-effects including confusion, hallucinations, ankle oedema and livedo reticularis

Selegiline

The history and pharmacology of selegiline are discussed in chapter 6. This chapter discusses its use as a symptomatic treatment both as monotherapy and adjuvant therapy in PD.

Monotherapy trials

The monotherapy trials with selegiline, discussed in chapter 6 when considering neuroprotective therapies, showed that it could delay the need for levodopa introduction by about nine months. The deterioration of patients after washout of selegiline suggested that this may have been due to a symptomatic effect. It can be argued that delaying levodopa for only nine months suggests a rather weak symptomatic effect. Most of the selegiline trials were placebo-controlled or combined selegiline with levodopa rather than comparing selegiline monotherapy with a dopamine agonist or levodopa alone, so no comparative data are available on true monotherapy. The UK PD MED trial will examine this issue with PD patients randomized between the three treatments and followed on an intention-to-treat basis.

Adjuvant trials

A recent five-year double-blind RCT in PD (n=163) compared selegiline combined with levodopa to levodopa alone. This showed that selegiline reduced the need for levodopa and reduced the decline in motor function. Furthermore, when the randomized medication was withdrawn at the end of five years, no deterioration in motor function was seen in those taking selegiline. This argues against any symptomatic effect of selegiline after this

length of time when used with levodopa and in favour of a neuroprotective effect.

> Selegiline can be used as an adjuvant to levodopa therapy

Selegiline adjuvant therapy was evaluated in trials in the mid-1980s. These were mainly small RCTs against placebo and suffered from being short-term and using a variety of different rating scales of motor impairments only. They showed that selegiline has a significant beneficial effect on motor impairments and that levodopa dose can be reduced, but whether or not this translates into worthwhile improvements in quality of life was not evaluated. There is a perception that selegiline is not as effective as the dopamine agonists, but no trials have compared adjuvant dopamine agonist therapy with selegiline. The PD MED trial will examine those PD patients on levodopa with motor complications who will be randomized between any dopamine agonist, any monoamine oxidase (MAO) B inhibitor, and any catechol-O-methyltransferase (COMT) inhibitor following them for at least five years and looking at quality of life and health economics outcomes.

> It is not known which form of adjuvant therapy (dopamine agonist, selegiline or COMT inhibitor) is superior

The results of adjuvant therapy trials with the novel oral fast-melt Zydis preparation of selegiline are just becoming available. In the largest of these to date, 163 patients with severe motor fluctuations (>3 hours 'off' time daily) were randomized to Zydis selegiline 1.25 mg/day, increasing after six weeks to 2.5 mg/day for six weeks or placebo. The therapeutic gain (treatment effect minus placebo effect) in 'off' time was 5.4% (~0.9 hours) on 1.25 mg/day and 9.0% (~1.4 hours) on 2.5 mg/day, both improvements being significant compared with placebo. Motor

Unified Parkinson's Disease Rating Scale (UPDRS) scores, both 'on' and 'off', were improved significantly on Zydis selegiline compared with placebo, and adverse events were acceptable.

> A new oral fast-melt preparation of selegiline is now available

Adverse effects

The adverse event profile of selegiline at any stage of PD is similar to that of the other dopamimetic therapies. Thus, nausea, vomiting, postural hypotension, confusion, hallucinations and insomnia can occur. The latter is often overlooked and can be associated with vivid dreams and nightmares even when selegiline is taken once-daily in the morning.

> Selegiline is prone to causing typical dopaminergic side-effects but particularly insomnia, vivid dreams and nightmares

COMT inhibitors

By blocking the metabolism of levodopa by the enzyme aromatic amino acid decarboxylase (AADC), predominantly in the gut wall, benserazide and carbidopa increase the bioavailability of levodopa two- to threefold and reduce peripheral side-effects. Despite the co-administration of an AADC inhibitor, only 5–10% of the orally administered levodopa crosses the blood–brain barrier. Much of the rest is metabolized to 3-O-methyldopa by the enzyme COMT, which was first described in 1958. It was hypothesized that blocking the actions of both COMT and AADC might further increase the bioavailability of levodopa (Figure 7.3, page 48).

Types of COMT inhibitors

The COMT inhibitors can be divided into two groups:

- *first generation COMT inhibitors* – these appeared in the 1960s and included pyrogallol, tropolones and 3,4-dihydroxy-2-methylpropiophenone (U-0521). These compounds suffered from weak or non-selective activity, poor bioavailability or high toxicity, but some did show promising enhancement of the effects of levodopa in animal models

- *second generation COMT inhibitors* – the structure of the second generation COMT inhibitors was first published by several groups in 1989 (Figure 9.1). These agents are di-substituted nitrocatechols which do not act in the gut to increase levodopa absorption. They seem to have a number of peripheral effects on levodopa metabolism resulting in a 30–50% increase in levodopa half-life and a 25–100% increase in the levodopa concentration versus time curve (area under the curve), but they do not increase the maximum plasma concentration of levodopa. More levodopa is, therefore, available for a longer period of time to cross the blood–brain barrier, in order to produce a more prolonged effect. Tolcapone also has a central effect which may at least in part account for its greater clinical efficacy. Of the second generation COMT inhibitors, tolcapone and entacapone are discussed in detail below. The clinical pharmacology of these agents is summarized in Table 9.2.

> By blocking COMT, entacapone and tolcapone increase the amount of levodopa reaching the brain

Tolcapone

Tolcapone was the first COMT inhibitor to be licensed for use in PD in the UK. Despite promising results in single-dose and chronic administration studies, it was withdrawn from European Commission countries in November 1998 after the reporting of six cases of hepatitis, two of which were fulminant and

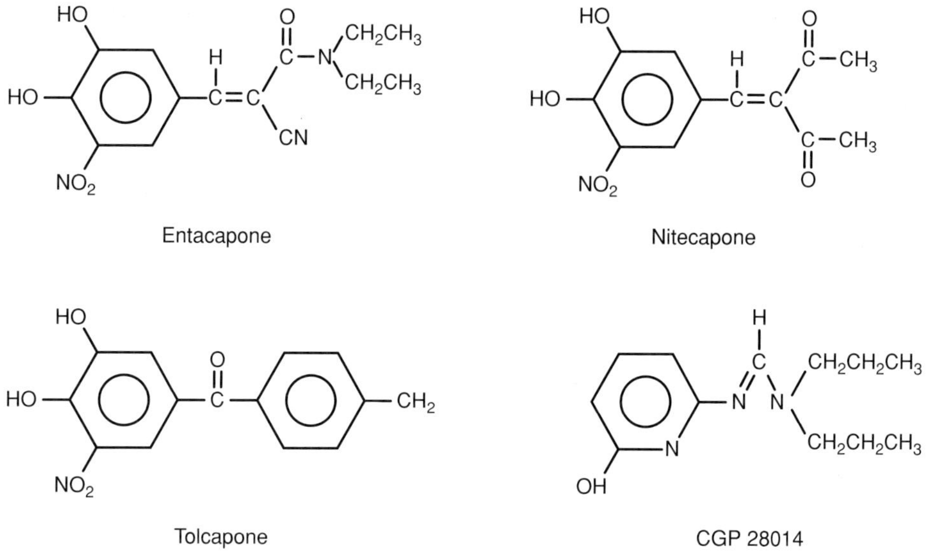

Figure 9.1
Chemical structure of the second generation COMT inhibitors

ultimately fatal. This was based on experience in 60,000 PD patients at the time. In the US, the Federal Drug Administration has not withdrawn the drug but the dose must be restricted to 100 mg tid and only increased to 200 mg tid in exceptional circumstances; liver enzyme monitoring has also been tightened. However, after reviewing the post-licensing clinical experience and trials with tolcapone in the US with a consensus panel including hepatologists, Olanow and colleagues concluded that:

- tolcapone is effective in PD
- irreversible liver injury is negligible with appropriate monitoring
- monitoring of liver function can be reduced after six months of treatment
- treatment should only stop if enzymes rise two to three times above the upper limit of normal.

The European regulatory authorities continue to review the experience with tolcapone annually and there is a possibility that it may be re-

Table 9.2
Clinical pharmacology of tolcapone and entacapone

Drug	Structure	Sites of action	T_{max} (h)	Half-life (h)	Dose frequency	Tablet doses (mg)	Clinical dose range (mg/day)
Entacapone	Nitrocatechol	Peripheral	0.4–0.9	0.3–0.4(α) 1.6–3.4(β)*	With every levodopa dose	200	400–1200
Tolcapone†	Nitrocatechol	Peripheral and central	0.9–2.0	2.0–3.0	tid	100 and 200	300–600

* two-phase model for elimination
† withdrawn from UK market in 1998

introduced in the UK. For this reason, further details on clinical trials with tolcapone will be briefly reviewed.

> Tolcapone was withdrawn from the European market in November 1998 because of several cases of fatal hepatic toxicity, but there is a possibility that it may be re-introduced in the UK

Clinical trials

The placebo-controlled studies with tolcapone were all double-blind trials but short-term, with the longest lasting 12 weeks. Most studies found significant reductions in 'off' time (treatment effect range 0.9–2.4 h/day) and levodopa dose (treatment effect range 67–251 mg/day). A few trials demonstrated significant benefits in UPDRS ADL or motor scores with tolcapone although this was probably due to insufficient patients being randomized in the studies (ie a false negative result). This is also suggested by the significant improvement in UPDRS activities of daily living (ADL) and motor scores in the larger and longer Waters *et al* study in patients before the onset of motor complications.

Two trials compared tolcapone directly with dopamine agonists as adjuvant therapy in PD. The bromocriptine-controlled study showed that tolcapone had similar effects on 'off' time and UPDRS motor and ADL scores, but it produced a significantly greater reduction in levodopa dose. The pergolide comparitor trial showed that the two drugs were very similar, although full publication of these results is awaited.

Adverse effects

Tolcapone generated typical dopaminergic adverse events, particularly dyskinesia. Diarrhoea was an unexpected side-effect which necessitated withdrawal in a significant number of patients. The reason for the diarrhoea remains unknown. During clinical trials, an increase in aspartate transaminase was found in only 1.7% of patients at 100 mg tid and in 3.1% at 200 mg tid. This necessitated the caveat in the Summary of Product Characteristics requiring liver function test monitoring. It also caused intensification in the yellow colour of the urine.

Entacapone

Only the results of placebo-controlled trials are available with entacapone. These studies generally lasted six months. Significant improvements in 'on' time (treatment effect range 1.0–2.1 h/day) and 'off' time (treatment effect range 1.3–1.5 h/day) were found. Significant reductions in levodopa dose occurred in all studies (treatment effect range 79–140 mg/day). Insufficient data are available on UPDRS ADL and motor scores to reach any firm conclusion about its effect on quality of life.

Adverse effects

Entacapone produced typical dopaminergic adverse events which could be reduced by levodopa dose reduction in most cases. It also caused diarrhoea and discoloration of urine similar to tolcapone. However, unlike tolcapone, no changes in liver function tests were found in the clinical trial programme or in post-marketing surveillance.

> Entacapone produces typical dopaminergic side-effects along with diarrhoea and yellow discoloration of urine

Clinical use

A Cochrane systematic review of tolcapone and entacapone adjuvant therapy is currently underway. Trials are underway in man to assess whether or not the addition of entacapone to small doses of levodopa is superior to larger doses of levodopa alone. However, the results of the equivalent study in MPTP-treated marmosets showed that dyskinesia developed just as quickly when entacapone was used as a levodopa-sparing agent.

Entacapone can be used as an adjuvant therapy to levodopa once motor complications have developed

No evidence is available on whether the addition of a dopamine agonist, MAO B inhibitor or entacapone is superior in a PD patient with motor complications taking levodopa. The PD MED trial will investigate this issue using quality of life and health economics outcomes.

It is not known which form of adjuvant therapy – dopamine agonist, selegiline or entacapone – is superior

Propranolol

In view of the well-known tremorigenic effect of adrenaline, the first β-adrenergic antagonist to be introduced – pronethalol – in 1963 was tested in a small number of parkinsonian patients with some beneficial results. Unfortunately, pronethalol was withdrawn due to carcinogenesis in mice but was replaced by propranolol. A number of studies examined the anti-tremor action of propranolol in PD in the late 1960s and early 1970s. In common with all the early studies in the condition, they generally suffered from the drawbacks of:

- a mixed sample of parkinsonism of different aetiologies
- small numbers
- the absence of a control arm
- the use of measures of motor impairment (eg accelerometry) which had little meaning in terms of ADL and quality of life.

However, these studies suggested that propranolol had a useful effect for both resting and postural tremor in parkinsonian syndromes, particularly if the dose could be titrated up to the range of 120–240 mg/day. Initial enthusiasm was dampened when a double-blind placebo-controlled study in 22 patients with PD showed statistically significant improvements in writing and circle-drawing with 120 mg/day propranolol, but no improvement in other measures of motor impairment, including tremor, or in 'total disability'.

More recently the long-acting preparation of propranolol has been evaluated in 10 patients with PD in a double-blind cross-over study which was not placebo-controlled but compared 160 mg/day long-acting propranolol with primidone 250 mg at night and clonazepam 4 mg/day. The latter agents were ineffective on tremor but generated significant adverse events. Long-acting propranolol reduced the mean amplitude of rest tremor by 70% and postural tremor by 50% without significant side-effects. Whether this is translated into significant benefit in terms of ADL or quality of life was not evaluated.

Propranolol can be used to reduce the amplitude of tremor in PD but it is unclear whether this improves quality of life

Further reading

Adler CH, Singer C, O'Brien C et al. Randomised placebo-controlled study of tolcapone in patients with fluctuating Parkinson disease treated with levodopa-carbidopa. Arch Neurol 1998; 55: 1089–95.

Assal F, Sphar L, Hadengue A et al. Tolcapone and fulminant hepatitis. Lancet 1998; 352: 958.

Axelrod J, Tomchick R. Enzymatic 0-methylation of epinephrine and other catechols. J Biol Chem 1958; 233: 702–5.

Baas H, Beiske AG, Ghika J et al. Catechol-0-methyl transferase inhibition with tolcapone reduces the wearing off phenomenon and levodopa requirements in fluctuating parkinsonian patients. J Neurol Neurosurg Psychiatry 1997; 63: 421–8.

Bonifati V, Meco G. New, selective catechol-0-methyltransferase inhibitors as therapeutic agents in Parkinson's disease. Pharmacol Ther 1999; 81: 1–36.

Deuschl G, Poewe W, Poepping M, The Celomen Study Group. Efficacy and safety of entacapone as an adjunctive to levodopa treatment in Parkinson's disease: experience from the Austrian-German six months study. Parkinsonism Relat Disord 1999; 5: S75.

Dupont E, Burgunder J, Findlay LJ et al. Tolcapone added to levodopa in stable parkinsonian patients: a double-blind placebo-controlled study. Mov Disord 1997; 12: 928–34.

Gilligan BS, Veale JL, Wodak J. Propranolol in the treatment of tremor. Med J Aust 1972; 1: 320–2.

Jenner P, Maratos E, Smith L, Jackson M. Correlation between L-dopa exposure and dyskinesia in MPTP-treated marmosets. Mov Disord 2000; 15(suppl 3): 19–20.

Koller WC, Herbster G. Adjuvant therapy of parkinsonian tremor. Arch Neurol 1987; 44: 921–3

Koller WC, Lees A, Morris J, Sterman A. A multicentre trial comparing the efficacy, tolerability, and safety of tolcapone versus pergolide in Parkinsons patients with motor fluctuations. Mov Disord 1998; 13(suppl 2): 52.

Kurth M, Adler C, St Hilaire M et al. Tolcapone improves motor function and reduces levodopa requirement in patients with Parkinson's disease experiencing motor fluctuations. Neurology 1997; 48: 81–7.

Larsen J, Boas J, Erdal J, The Norwegian-Danish Study Group. Does selegiline modify the progression of early Parkinson's disease? Results from a five-year study. Eur J Neurol 1999; 6: 539–47.

Marsden CD, Parkes JD, Rees JE. Propranolol in Parkinson's Disease. Lancet 1974; 2: 410.

Olanow CW. Tolcapone and hepatotoxic effects. Tasmar Advisory Panel. Arch Neurol 2000; 57: 263–7.

The Parkinson Study Group. Entacapone improves motor fluctuations in levodopa-treated Parkinson's disease patients. Ann Neurol 1997; 42: 747–55.

Rajput AH, Martin W, Saint-Hilaire MH et al. Tolcapone improves motor function in parkinsonian patients with the wearing off phenomenon: a double-blind, placebo-controlled, multicentre trial. Neurology 1997; 49: 1066–71.

Rinne U, Larsen JP, Siden A et al. Entacapone enhances the response to levodopa in parkinsonian patients with motor fluctuations. Neurology 1998; 51: 1309–14.

Ruottinen HM, Rinne UK. Entacapone prolongs levodopa response in a one month double-blind study in parkinsonian patients with levodopa related fluctuations. J Neurol Neurosurg Psychiatry 1996; 60: 36–40.

Sagar H, Brooks D, UK-Irish Entacapone Study Group. The UK-Irish double-blind study of entacapone in Parkinson's disease. Mov Disord 2000; 15(suppl 3): 135.

Schwab R, Chafetz M. Kemadrin in the treatment of parkinsonism. Neurology 1955; 5: 273–7.

Shellenberger MK, Clarke A, Donoghue S. Zydis selegiline reduces 'off' time and improves symptoms in patients with Parkinson's disease. Mov Disord 2000; 15(suppl 3): 116.

The Tolcapone Study Group. Efficacy and tolerability of tolcapone compared with bromocriptine in levodopa-treated parkinsonian patients. Mov Disord 1999; 14: 38–44.

Verhagen-Metman L, Del Dotto P, van den Munckhof P et al. Amantadine as a treatment for dyskinesias and motor fluctuations in Parkinson's disease. Neurology 1998; 50: 1323–6.

Waters CH, Kurth M, Bailey P et al. Tolcapone in stable Parkinson's disease: efficacy and safety of long-term treatment. Neurology 1997; 49: 665–71.

10. Medical management – specific problems

Depression
Psychosis
Dementia
Constipation
Micturition (urinary) disturbance
Sleep disturbance
Postural instability and falls

Depression

Depression is a significant clinical problem in patients with idiopathic Parkinson's disease (PD). The precise scale of the condition is unclear.

Prevalence and quality of life

The prevalence of depression in studies of parkinsonian patients varies widely, ranging between 4% and 90% depending on the criteria used for diagnosis and whether studies were community- or hospital-based. In 1992, the mean prevalence of depression was calculated to be 40% in 26 studies. In a more recent Norwegian community-based study, depression was found in 26% of patients; in a similar study in North Wales, it was found in 64% of patients with PD referred to a geriatric service and in 34% of their carers.

Depression affects 40% of patients with PD

The impact of depression on the lives of patients with PD has further been underlined in recent years by quality of life studies. For example, the Norwegian community-based study examined quality of life in 233 patients with PD using the Nottingham Health Profile. It revealed that 54% of the reduction in quality of life could be explained by depression, sleep problems, low Schwab and England score (disease-specific ADL scale), low Unified Parkinson's Disease Rating Scale (UPDRS) motor score, and levodopa dose. Similarly, the Global Parkinson's Disease Survey (co-sponsored by the United Kingdom Parkinson's Disease Society) examined quality of life using the PDQ-39 questionnaire in more than 1,000 patients in six countries, which revealed that more than 40% of the reduction in quality of life was explained by depression compared with 17% for Hoehn and Yahr stage (page 24) and medication.

40% of reduced quality of life in PD is explained by depression compared with only 17% for motor impairments

The current practice of many clinicians when assessing a patient with PD in the clinic is to concentrate on motor impairments and the patient's response to therapy. Quality of life data demonstrate that depression accounts for more reduction in quality of life than motor impairment, suggesting that this attitude to clinical assessment is inadequate. We must develop ways of routinely looking for depression in all PD patients.

The prevalence of depression in PD is greater than occurs in other chronic disorders with similar levels of disability. This, combined with the occurrence of depression before the onset of motor disability and the lack of correlation between its severity and motor disability, suggests that a significant proportion of depression in PD is endogenous and perhaps part of the disease process rather than a reaction to the disability.

Depression may be part of the disease process of PD rather than a reaction to the disability

Pathophysiology

The neural mechanism of depression in PD is unknown. It is tempting to suggest that dopamine depletion is the cause, since this is the underlying pathology of PD, reserpine (which depletes dopamine from storage vesicles) causes depression, and depression can develop during PD patients' 'off' periods. However, treatment to reverse dopamine deficiency, such as levodopa, does not reverse depression, despite increasing mesolimbic dopamine. Noradrenaline and 5-hydroxytryptamine are also depleted in PD and may play a part in the genesis of depression.

Rating scales

Many depression rating scales have been used in PD, including the:

- Beck Depression Inventory (BDI)
- Hamilton Depression Rating Scale (HDRS)
- Hospital Anxiety and Depression Scale (HADS)
- Montgomery and Asberg Depression Rating Scale (MADRS).

Systematic comparison of these scales has not been undertaken in PD, but most studies in the past have used the BDI both as a screening tool and to monitor treatment.

Treatment

Once depression has been identified, some measure of its severity is needed to judge the level of therapeutic intervention required. In a study of 40 parkinsonian patients, only four fulfilled the International Classification of Disease (ICD)-9 criteria for 'caseness'. Thus, many patients may have a very mild depressive syndrome which may require pharmacotherapy, whereas others may need formal psychiatric evaluation and even more aggressive treatment such as electroconvulsive therapy (ECT).

Pharmacotherapy

The value of pharmacotherapy for depression in PD has been poorly studied. A systematic review of the literature up to June 1993 found 12 randomized controlled trials of antidepressant therapy in PD, but five of these examined the antidepressant action of the antiparkinsonian drug selegiline. The remaining studies were placebo-controlled and examined tricyclic antidepressants. The studies were small, used vague and varied outcome measures, and were short-term, so it proved impossible to draw any conclusions about the efficacy and safety of this class of antidepressant in PD. The selective serotonin reuptake inhibitors (SSRIs) sertraline and citalopram have undergone limited trials in depression in PD, but these were also small studies with small positive effects requiring confirmation in larger trials. The balance between efficacy and adverse events is a particular issue with antidepressant therapy in this condition. Case reports of worsening parkinsonian symptoms with SSRI treatment have appeared, and in one survey 43% of clinicians were concerned that this was a serious problem with this class of antidepressant.

> Clinical trials of antidepressant therapy in PD are few and of poor quality

From a questionnaire study of antidepressant prescribing habits of members of the North American Parkinson Study Group, it was estimated that 26% of patients were depressed and receiving antidepressant therapy. SSRIs were used as first-line treatment by 51% of clinicians and the tricyclics by 41%. The former were chosen because of their better side-effect profile and efficacy, whereas the tricyclics were selected to help with sleep and because of greater experience with their use. It was concluded that uncertainties remain regarding antidepressant use and that a controlled clinical trial would be of value.

> There is no firm evidence of deterioration in parkinsonism with SSRI class drugs

In the absence of trial evidence, no guidelines for antidepressant use can be provided

Electroconvulsive therapy (ECT)

ECT may be required for patients with severe depression in PD. This therapy can be very successful both for depression and the associated severe psychomotor retardation which can add to the severity of the patient's motor disability.

Psychosis

This is a spectrum ranging from mild illusions, visual hallucinations and vivid dreams, which patients will often choose to tolerate, through to frank psychosis with paranoid delusions and upsetting visual hallucinations. Precise prevalence figures are variable depending on the clinical context and the medication the patient is taking.

Pathophysiology

Psychosis is often caused by underlying Lewy body dementia or the patient's medication. Even relatively young patients can develop psychosis when they first start medication, most commonly with a dopamine agonist. The reason why they are so sensitive is not known. When psychosis develops in later disease, without any recent change in medication, it is often the harbinger of dementia and the need for nursing home placement may not be too far off.

The pathophysiology of psychosis is not fully understood. Dopaminergic pathways to the limbic system and cortex are involved in PD and may take part in generating such symptoms. Other degenerate catecholaminergic pathways, particularly those using 5-hydroxytryptamine (5-HT) as a transmitter, may be involved.

Treatment

The first step in the management of psychosis is to decide with the patient and carer whether or not the symptoms are sufficiently distressing to require intervention. Many patients are reasonably happy to continue with occasional formed visual illusions of people or animals sitting next to them. In this situation, no change in treatment may be necessary. Any precipitating infection or dehydration must be treated. The next step is to withdraw any recently commenced antiparkinsonian medication which may be the precipitant. Thereafter, minor agents such as anticholinergics, amantadine and selegiline should be withdrawn. This may only have a small impact on the patient's motor function. Dopamine agonists and levodopa should then be reduced cautiously, accepting a significant fall in mobility. This is often the point at which nursing home admission is required.

An alternative approach at any point in the above scheme is to consider adding an anti-psychotic agent. The older generation agents (eg haloperidol) block dopaminergic transmission in motor pathways so the patient's motor function deteriorates. This led to the search for a modern anti-psychotic which did not cause deterioration in motor function. Quite a number of small trials have now shown that the atypical neuroleptic clozapine, which is mainly a D_4 rather than a D_2 receptor antagonist, can reduce psychotic symptoms. However, neutropenia occurs in 1–2% of patients, so detailed monitoring is required. The absence of a licence for this indication in the UK also limits its use to a named-patient basis within large centres which have a psychiatrist accustomed to using the drug. Subsequent studies with risperidone and olanzapine have shown that motor function does deteriorate with these agents. The early work with quetiapine is more hopeful but controlled studies have yet to be reported. The 5-HT_3 receptor antagonist ondansetron is used as an antiemetic in the oncology field. Some small trials have suggested that it may be useful in parkinsonian psychosis without interfering with motor function. Further work is required before this expensive drug can be recommended. The management of psychosis in PD is outlined in Table 10.1.

Dementia

Lewy body dementia may present with the clinical features of PD along with a subsequent dementia or primarily with a dementia with associated, and often subtle, extrapyramidal features. The characteristic features of this type of dementia are:

- the presence of visual hallucinations
- a fluctuating course, often with lucid intervals
- extrapyramidal features suggesting PD.

> Dementia presents with fluctuating cognitive decline, visual hallucinations and often, but not always, a parkinsonian syndrome

Impairment of short-term memory is not perhaps as prominent as in Alzheimer's disease or multiple infarct dementia in the early stages. Behavioural disturbance, often with frontal features such as lack of judgment, inattention and indecisiveness, can occur. These features are commonly associated with psychosis.

By the time a Lewy body dementia has been formally diagnosed, the patient is usually suffering from psychotic features which require the management strategy outlined in Table 10.1. This will only reduce the symptoms of the disorder with no effect on the underlying condition and its progression.

Table 10.1
Management of psychosis in PD

1. Treat any precipitating infection or dehydration
2. Slowly reduce, then withdraw, anticholinergics, selegiline, amantadine and dopamine agonists using the 'last one in, first one out' rule
3. If absolutely necessary reduce levodopa slowly and accept deteriorating mobility
4. Consider adding a new generation anti-psychotic (eg quetiapine) or ondansetron
5. Prevent complications of immobility (eg heparin)

> The management measures suggested for treating psychosis can be useful for dementia in PD

Recently, early studies with the new acetylcholinesterase inhibitors, licensed for use in Alzheimer's disease, have been performed in the hope that this class of drug can slow the progression of Lewy body dementia. The results presented so far suggest that they may be able to improve some aspects of cognition and even a few psychotic symptoms without deterioration in motor function. There had been concern that by increasing levels of acetylcholine in the striatum, patients' motor function would decline; it will be recalled that anticholinergics are used to treat the condition. Further larger-scale and longer trials are now required in this area.

> Small trials with the anticholinesterase agents donepezil and rivastigmine have shown promising results PD

Constipation

Constipation in PD is extremely common, even early in the course of the disease. It is probably caused by direct involvement of the myenteric plexus in the pathology of the condition, as Lewy bodies are found in the gut wall. Management should follow a pragmatic policy of increased fluids and fibre initially, leading to the use of laxatives individually and then in combination depending on the patient's response.

> Constipation should initially be treated with increased fluids, fruit and fibre. If therapeutic trials of several laxatives used independently fails, the a combination of agents from different classes should be used

Micturition (urinary) disturbance

Severe micturition (urinary) problems, particularly early in the course of the disease, raise the prospect of an alternative diagnosis, often multiple system atrophy (page 23), or concurrent conditions such as prostatism. The physical limitations of the patient's motor disabilities must also be considered – he or she may not be able to reach a toilet in time.

> Early bladder disturbance suggests an alternative diagnosis such as MSA, or another problem such as prostatism. Physicians should ensure the patient's poor mobility is not the primary cause of incontinence

However, a significant proportion of patients develop mild to moderate detrusor hyper-reflexia due to central abnormalities in the pontine micturition centre. These do respond to peripheral antimuscarinic agents such as oxybutynin and tolterodine, which are generally well tolerated.

> Moderate detrusor hyper-reflexia can be controlled with oxybutynin or tolterodine

Sleep disturbance

Sleep disturbance is very common in PD, occurring in up to 98% of patients. Specific conditions account for a proportion of these cases. For example:

- Restless Legs Syndrome (RLS), which can be the harbinger of PD or can occur in association with it (page 19)
- Rapid Eye Movement (REM) Sleep Behaviour Disorder (RBD), which is seen in some PD patients and manifests as purposeful nocturnal motor activity during REM sleep in keeping with dream enactment. Normally, we are atonic during REM sleep, but this does not occur in RBD. Patients are often violent and cry out during these periods. Whether the condition is caused by the underlying pathology of PD or this combined with treatment is uncertain (page 20).

However, many patients have less specific symptomatology such as:

- periodic limb movements
- myoclonic jerks
- a return of tremor which disturbs and, thus, fragments sleep.

> Some patients have specific problems such as RLS and REM sleep behaviour disorder, but most have non-specific disorders such as periodic limb movements

Management

Management relies on good sleep hygiene to avoid inverting the sleep–wake cycle; this involves ensuring regular bedtimes and not allowing naps during the day. Short-acting benzodiazepines such as Temazepam can be useful. Improved treatment of daytime motor problems seems to help nocturnal difficulties. The specific treatment for RLS is either a modified-release levodopa preparation taken at night or a dopamine agonist such as cabergoline in view of its long half-life. RBD should be treated with clonazepam 0.5–2.0 mg at night and usually has a good response. Table 10.2 summarizes the management of sleep disturbance in PD.

Table 10.2
Points to note for managing sleep disturbance in PD

- Start with good sleep hygiene, ensuring regular bedtimes and no daytime naps
- Improve the treatment of daytime mobility problems
- Specific conditions may require specific treatments, eg:
  - RLS with either modified-release levodopa or a long-acting dopamine agonist such as cabergoline
  - REM sleep behaviour disorder with clonazepam
- Non-specific conditions can be treated with short-acting benzodiazepines, such as Temazepam

---

Postural instability and falls

These usually occur late in the course of PD and are difficult to treat, responding poorly to increases in antiparkinsonian medication. Falls not infrequently lead to fractures which can be life-threatening but at least reduce quality of life and increase the costs of care. This has recently been recognized in the National Service Framework for the Elderly. Instability can be demonstrated by the 'pull test' in which the patient stands with his or her feet slightly apart and, after a warning from the examiner, is pulled sharply backwards at the shoulders. If the patient falls uncontrollably backwards into the examiner's hands, the test is positive.

> Falls early in the course of a parkinsonian syndrome suggest progressive supranuclear palsy

Management should consist of a multidisciplinary assessment of the patient, preferably within his or her own home, by an experienced team of physiotherapists and occupational therapists. Strategies such as walking aids (eg sticks, frames) may be required and certain flooring surfaces such as thick pile carpet may have to be removed.

> Falls in PD respond poorly to increases in medication – patients may need walking aids and other adaptations

> Multidisciplinary assessment, preferably in the patient's home, should be performed

Ultimately, despite the best medical and paramedical therapy efforts, recurrent falls can be the final straw that lead to residential care placement.

Further reading

Andersen J, Aabro E, Gulmann N et al. Anti-depressive treatment in Parkinson's disease. A controlled trial of the effect of nortriptyline in patients with Parkinson's disease treated with L-DOPA. Acta Neurol Scand 1980; 62: 210–9.

Beck AT, Ward CH, Mendelson M et al. An inventory for measuring depression. Arch Gen Psychiatry 1961; 4: 561–71.

Brown RG, MacCarthy B. Psychiatric morbidity in patients with Parkinson's disease. Psychol Med 1990; 20: 77–87.

Cummings JL. Depression and Parkinson's disease: a review. Am J Psychiatry 1992; 4: 443–54.

Fernandez HH, Friedman JH, Jacques C, Rosenfeld M. Quetiapine for the treatment of drug-induced psychosis in Parkinson's disease. Mov Disord 1999; 14: 484–7.

Findley L, Peto V, Pugner K et al. The impact of Parkinson's disease on quality of life: results of a research survey in the UK. Mov Disord 2000; 15(suppl 3): 179.

Friedberg G, Zoldan J, Weizman A, Melamed E. Parkinson Psychosis Rating Scale: a practical instrument for grading psychosis in Parkinson's disease. Clin Neuropharmacol 1998; 21: 280–4.

Hauser RA, Zesiewicz TA. Sertraline for the treatment of depression in Parkinson's disease. Mov Disord 1997; 12: 756–9.

Jimenez-Jimenez FJ, Tejeiro J, Martinez-Junquera G et al. Parkinsonism exacerbated by paroxetine. Neurology 1994; 44: 2406.

Karlsen KH, Larsen JP, Tandberg E, Maeland JG. Influence of clinical and demographic variables on quality of life in patients with Parkinson's disease. J Neurol, Neurosurg Psychiatry 1999; 66: 431–5.

Klaassen T, Verhey FRJ, Sneijders GHJM et al. Treatment of depression in Parkinson's disease: a meta-analysis. J Neuropsychiatry Clin Neurosci 1995; 7: 281–6.

Laitinen L. Desipramine in treatment of Parkinson's disease. A placebo-controlled study. Acta Neurol Scand 1969; 45: 109–13.

Lees AJ, Blackburn NA, Campbell VL. The nighttime problems of Parkinson's disease. Clin Neuropharmacol 1988; 11: 512–9

Mayeux R. Mental state. In: Koller W, ed. Handbook of Parkinson's Disease. New York: Marcel Dekker, 1987: 127–43.

Mayeux R. Depression and dementia in Parkinson's disease. In: Marsden CD, Fahn S, eds. Movement disorders. London: Butterworth, 1982: 75–95.

Meara J, Mitchelmore E, Hobson P. Use of the GDS-15 geriatric depression scale as a screening instrument for depressive symptomatology in patients with Parkinson's disease and their carers in the community. Age Ageing 1999; 28: 35–8.

Molho ES, Factor SA. Worsening of motor features of parkinsonism with olanzapine. Mov Disord 1999; 14: 1014–6.

Richard IH, Kurlan R, Group PS. A survey of antidepressant drug use in Parkinson's disease. Neurology 1997; 49: 1168–70.

Strang RR. Imipramine in treatment of parkinsonism: a double-blind placebo study. BMJ 1965; 2: 33–4.

Tandberg E, Larsen JP, Aarsland D, Cummings JL. The occurrence of depression in Parkinson's disease. A community-based study. *Arch Neurol* 1996; **53:** 175–9.

Wermuth L, Sorensen P, Timm S *et al.* Depression in idiopathic Parkinson's disease treated with citalopram. A placebo-controlled trial. *Nordic J Psychiatry* 1998; **52:** 163–9.

11. Surgical management

Functional neurosurgery
Intracerebral grafting

Functional neurosurgery
Brief history

With the lack of adequate therapy for idiopathic Parkinson's disease (PD) and the evolution of safe neurosurgery, various surgical approaches to the condition were attempted in the 1930s and 1940s. Lesions were placed in the corticospinal pathway in the spinal cord, the dentate nucleus of the cerebellum and the premotor cortex, with little beneficial effect and considerable morbidity and mortality. In 1952, Cooper ligated the anterior choroidal artery of a patient with PD during another operation. The beneficial effects of this procedure led to further operations with variable results, but it did encourage others to explore lesioning of the outflow pathways from the globus pallidus. The mixed success of such procedures was probably due to poor localization techniques. This improved with the availability of accurate three-dimensional targeting using stereotaxis, which had originally been introduced by Spiegel and Wycis in 1946. The breakthrough came in 1960 when Leksell's group found that lesions placed in the posteroventral portion of the medial segment of the globus pallidus produced significant benefits in parkinsonian symptoms.

The dramatic success of levodopa in the 1960s then quashed further surgical development. However, the poor effects of levodopa on tremor left the way clear for thalamotomy, which was found to be more effective for tremor than the other features of the condition.

It was only in the early 1990s that Laitinen returned to posteroventral pallidotomy for more severe disease with associated motor complications which were unresponsive to pharmacotherapy. Since then, there has been a dramatic increase in the interest in functional neurosurgery for PD.

> Surgery is appropriate for a small minority of patients with PD

Rationale

The functional anatomy of the basal ganglia was outlined in chapter 3 and is reprised in Figure 11.1. In essence, movement is controlled by a pathway which passes from the premotor cortex through the striatum (putamen and caudate) and globus pallidus to the thalamus, and then back to the supplementary motor cortex. Activity in this loop is modulated by the substantia nigra, which acts like a motor car accelerator, and the subthalamic nucleus (STN), which acts like a brake. In PD, the nigra is defective, so the accelerator fails to work and the patient slows down. Following a stroke (usually an infarct) involving the STN, the brake is lost and the patient develops contralateral hemiballismus/hemichorea syndrome.

On the assumption that the 'accelerator' and 'brake' pathways work separately in a constant equilibrium (unlike a motor vehicle), a logical approach to the treatment of PD (in which the 'accelerator' is lost) is to switch off the 'brake'. More correctly, this means reducing the overactivity in the glutamatergic pathway from the STN to the globus pallidus pars medialis (GPM) and/or reducing the overactivity in the gabaminergic pathway from the GPM to the thalamus.

Reducing the activity of a pathway can be achieved by either lesioning it or overstimulating it so that it switches off physiologically (depolarization block). Lesioning is most commonly performed by stereotactic thermocoagulation, in which an electrode is accurately targeted through a burr

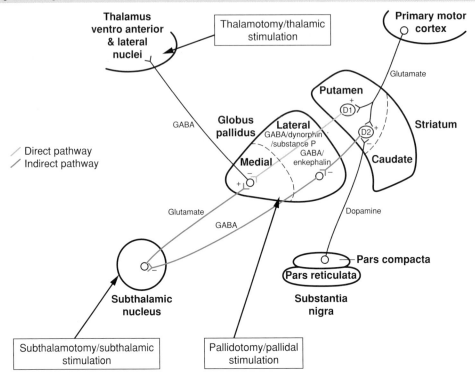

Figure 11.1
Sites of action of functional neurosurgical techniques. + = excitatory neurotransmitter; − = inhibitory neurotransmitter

hole in the skull to the site in question using magnetic resonance imaging (MRI) or computed tomography; a current is then passed through the electrode tip which heats up to a set temperature for a carefully judged period (Figure 11.2). Stimulation is achieved using

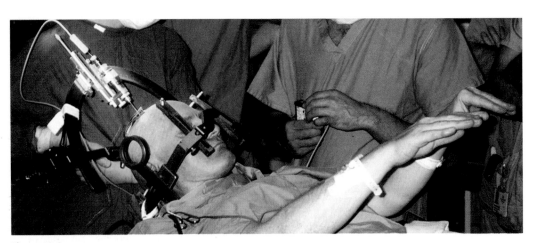

Figure 11.2
Stereostatic pallidotomy. Reproduced with permission from Mrs R Mitchell

similar technology to a cardiac pacemaker (Figure 11.3). An electrode is placed in the target using MRI stereotaxy which is then connected, via wiring tunnelled under the skin, to a 'pacing' box (pulse generator) placed under the anterior chest wall skin. The latter can then be programmed through the intact skin with an external probe connected to a computer. This method is often referred to as 'deep brain stimulation' (DBS).

Improved understanding of the pathophysiology of PD has led to the development of new surgical procedures in recent years

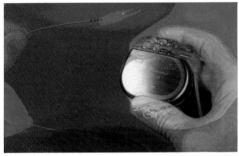

Figure 11.3
Pulse generator and stimulator tip. Courtesy of Medtronic

Pallidotomy

Posteroventral pallidotomy (PVP) was re-introduced by Laitinen in 1992 after Leksell's original work. There followed a dramatic increase in interest in the procedure with numerous groups publishing the results of their own case series. A recent review of this work, performed by the University of Birmingham Clinical Trials Unit as part of a grant application, revealed 68 reports of case series and trials which included about 2,324 patients with PD (this may be an overestimate because of multiple publication). Only four controlled trials of pallidotomy are known, usually against deferred surgery. No up-to-date systematic review of these data is available although a number of reviews have appeared. The fact that more than 2,300 patients can undergo a novel surgical procedure with very few being included in randomized controlled trials to establish its effectiveness and safety is surely a sad indictment of the lack of research planning in modern healthcare systems!

Most series have shown that the main benefit of PVP is in reducing contralateral dyskinesias, both choreoathetoid and dystonic (Table 11.1). Minor ipsilateral improvements in dyskinesia usually fade over the first few years following the operation. Motor impairments (usually

Table 11.1
Efficacy and safety of various forms of functional neurosurgery for PD

Outcome	Posteroventral pallidotomy	Thalamotomy (VIM nucleus)	Bilateral thalamic stimulation (VIM nucleus)	Bilateral STN stimulation	Bilateral pallidal stimulation
Dyskinesia	Contralateral +++	0	0	++	+
Tremor	Contralateral +	Contralateral +	+++	+	+
'Off' period motor impairment	+++	NA	0	+++	+++
'On' period motor impairment	0	NA	0	+	NA
Activities of daily living	++	NA	0	+++	+++
Medication	⇑⇑	⇒	⇒	⇓⇓	⇓
Morbidity	5%	5%	5%	NA	NA
Mortality	2%	NA	0%	NA	NA

+ = positive effect; 0 = no effect; NA = not available; ⇑ = increased; ⇒ = unchanged; ⇓ = decreased; VIM = ventrointermediate nucleus measured as Unified Parkinson's Disease Rating Score motor score) in the 'on' phase hardly change after the procedure, but there is generally a significant improvement in 'off' phase impairment bilaterally, which leads to an improvement in activities of daily living (ADL). There are few long-term studies of PVP, but the beneficial effects on contralateral dyskinesia, 'off' period motor impairments and ADL have been maintained in some series for about four years. Medication is often increased after PVP to treat underlying disease progression since dyskinesia has improved following the operation.

Bilateral PVP has been explored by only a few groups, usually as a staged procedure with the second operation weeks or months after the first. However, dysphagia and dysphonia are common side-effects which are likely to reduce the popularity of bilateral operations.

Most surgeons target the pallidum for PVP using one of the following techniques:

- macrostimulation via the lesioning electrode to test whether they are too near the optic tract or internal capsule
- micro-electrode recording with special fine electrodes to record the activity within the structures they pass through as the cannula is inserted.

Despite these precautions, a small number of patients develop visual field defects or hemiparesis after the procedure and intracerebral haemorrhage can occur with any technique (Figure 11.4). The risk of serious disability from the operation is generally quoted at around 5% and mortality at 2%. Limited evidence is available from one review of PVP to suggest that using microelectrode recording may increase mortality.

Pallidotomy has been re-introduced to reduce contralateral dyskinesia and 'off'-period motor impairments by allowing an increase in medication

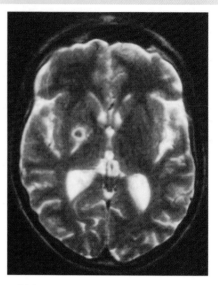

Figure 11.4
T2 weighted MRI scan two days after posteroventral pallidotomy showing the extent of oedema and the lesion

Subthalamotomy

An alternative to lesioning the overactive STN–GPM pathway in the pallidum is to target the much smaller STN itself – the technique of subthalamotomy. However, there has been concern that spontaneous lesions in this area, caused most commonly by strokes, lead to a hemichorea/hemiballismus syndrome. Research on the 1-methyl-4-phenyl-1,2,3,6-tetrahydropyridine (MPTP) primate model of PD showed that STN lesions could be achieved safely with little, if any, involuntary movements developing as a result of the operation. Several groups have recently started to examine the value of this procedure in patients with PD but insufficient data are available at present to judge its effectiveness and safety.

Thalamotomy

Traditionally, the ventrointermediate nucleus (VIM) of the thalamus has been the target for neurosurgical intervention. This nucleus is part of an oscillating circuit involving the cerebellum which may generate parkinsonian rest tremor. Lesions of the VIM nucleus can achieve abolition of tremor for many patients and this is frequently long-lasting, but little if any benefit results on rigidity, hypokinesia and bradykinesia. The trial reports from the early days of thalamotomy development do not allow accurate assessment of its effects or safety. However, modern experience suggests that more than 90% of patients will have a worthwhile reduction in tremor with long-term benefit. Morbidity is similar to PVP at around 5%. Dysarthria is the most frequent complication, particularly after bilateral operations.

> Thalamotomy has been used for many years to alleviate severe tremor in PD

Thalamic stimulation

The concept of DBS was introduced by Benabid and colleagues from Grenoble in the late 1980s. It was initially used to stimulate the VIM nucleus of the thalamus, thereby improving severe parkinsonian tremor. Limited uncontrolled studies have shown that clinically meaningful tremor reduction occurs in 85% of cases, a figure close to that achieved by thalamotomy. Follow-up has extended for three years with a suggestion that tolerance develops and that stimulation parameters need to be increased over time. No improvement in the other features of PD or dyskinesia occurs with VIM thalamic stimulation.

Dysarthria, imbalance and paraesthesia can occur with this technique but improve with decreased stimulation voltage. Unlike thalamotomy, bilateral implantation of thalamic stimulators does not seem to increase morbidity. In addition to the significant risk of intracerebral haemorrhage, stimulation brings its own unique risks of cable breaks and disconnections, local infection, battery failure and the need for replacement, reprogramming and significantly greater cost.

Subthalamic stimulation

Having pioneered the development of thalamic stimulation, the Grenoble group moved on to the STN. The group's success with this technique is such that most surgery for PD in France now uses this methodology. Bilateral implantation is usually performed during the same procedure (Figures 11.5 and 11.6).

No randomized controlled trial of STN stimulation versus deferred surgery or even chronic apomorphine infusion has been performed. The small case series published to date suggest that this procedure can improve 'off'-period motor impairments (UPDRS motor scores) and ADL (UPDRS ADL scores), which allows a reduction in medication and thus less dyskinesia. Too few operations have been performed to assess its safety or its benefits in the long-term. The cost of the operation itself and the hardware can amount to about £20,000 for bilateral stimulation. At present, insufficient information is available to perform a cost-

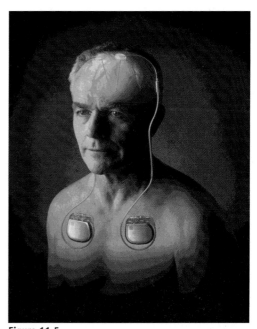

Figure 11.5
Bilateral implantation of subthalamic stimulators.
Courtesy of Medtronic

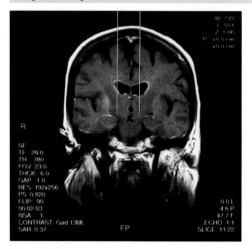

Figure 11.6
T1 weighted MRI scan after insertion of bilateral STN stimulators. Courtesy of Mrs R Mitchell

benefit analysis for the procedure. The Medical Research Council in the UK has part-funded with the Parkinson's Disease Society a trial of STN stimulation versus best medical practice which will include assessment of quality of life and health economics for 10 years postoperation (PD SURG Trial).

> Bilateral subthalamic nucleus stimulation is under evaluation and may reduce dyskinesia, improve 'off'-period motor implications and activities of daily living with a decrease in medication

Pallidal stimulation

Bilateral pallidal stimulation is still in its infancy, with very few published reports even of small case series. This early work and a single small randomized comparison of STN with pallidal stimulation suggests that it is as effective as STN stimulation in reducing 'off' period motor impairment and disability but medication reduction is less with the pallidal target.

Intracerebral grafting

The possibility of transplanting embryonic dopaminergic neurones into the striatum to

relieve symptoms of PD was first explored in the early 1980s by Bjorklund and Dunnett in the 6-hydroxydopamine rat model of the condition. They showed that the implanted cells survived and produced synaptic contacts with the host, which allowed some functional recovery.

The earliest trial of human fetal grafts in four patients with PD by Lindvall's team in Sweden was not encouraging, probably because of poor graft survival as evidenced by low fluorodopa uptake shown on positron emission tomography (PET) imaging (page 30). In a more recent cohort of patients, the Swedish group has had more success with mean increases in fluorodopa uptake of 68% 12 months after surgery. This was accompanied by improvements in motor impairments and, in one case, the ability to withdraw levodopa completely. In the single postmortem on a patient 18 months after such a graft, 10% of the putamen was found to be reinnervated. More recently in a trial of implantation versus, controversially, sham surgery in North America (n=40), a prohibitive amount of dyskinesia and dystonia developed which had not been seen in the Swedish studies.

Thus, the small number of case series published so far do not allow thorough assessment of the efficacy and safety of this technique. Further development will be hampered by the need for fetal midbrain cells. At present, four aborted human fetuses are used for each putamen; this presents considerable ethical and practical problems. This may be overcome by using stem cells or genetically engineered cells. Experiments in rats have shown that it is possible to grow host fibroblast cells taken from skin biopsies in tissue culture, transfect them with the gene for tyrosine hydroxylase, then transplant colonies of cells manufacturing levodopa into the 6-hydroxydopamine-treated host which generate significant functional recovery. However, translating early successes in the rat to patients with PD is proving to be a significant leap.

> Intracerebral grafting is under evaluation but further work is needed on the source of dopaminergic cells

Further reading

Aziz TZ, Peggs D, Sambrook MA, Crossman AR. Lesions of the subthalamic nucleus for the alleviation of 1-methyl-4-phenyl-1,2,3,6-tetrahydropyridine (MPTP)-induced parkinsonism in the primate. *Mov Disord* 1991; **6**: 288–92.

Fahn S. Double-blind controlled trial of embryonic dopaminergic tissue transplants in advanced Parkinson's disease. *Mov Disord* 2000; **15**(suppl 3): 7–8.

Gregory R, Bowen J. Posteroventral pallidotomy for advanced Parkinson's disease: a systematic review. *Neurol Reviews Int* 1999; **3**: 8–12.

Kordower JH, Freeman TB, Snow BJ *et al*. Neuropathological evidence of graft survival and striatal reinnervation after the transplantation of fetal mesenceaphalic tissue in a patient with Parkinson's disease. *N Engl J Med* 1995; **27**: 1118–24.

Lindvall O, Rechncrona S, Brundin P *et al*. Human fetal dopamine neurones grafted into the striatum in two patients with Parkinson's disease. *Arch Neurol* 1989; **46**: 615–31.

Shimohama S, Fisher LJ, Gage FH. Intracerebral grafting of genetically modified cells. *Adv Neurol* 1993; **60**: 744–8.

Wenning GK, Odin P, Morrish P *et al*. Short-and long-term survival and function of unilateral intrastriatal dopaminergic grafts in Parkinson's disease. *Ann Neurol* 1997; **42**: 95–107.

12. Supportive management

Paramedical therapies
Parkinson's Disease Nurse Specialists

Despite optimal medical and occasionally surgical therapy, patients with idiopathic Parkinson's disease (PD) suffer increasing disability and handicap due to the disease. This leads to reduced quality of life for both the patient and his or her carer, and increased costs for the family and the country as a whole. Earlier chapters have discussed the need for further work on issues such as depression and dementia particularly when motor function has been treated as far as possible. However, there is a potential for improving handicap and quality of life, and possibly reducing costs, using alternative interventions such as paramedical therapies and PD Nurse Specialists (PDNSs).

Paramedical therapies

It is generally accepted that rehabilitation is best provided as part of a multidisciplinary team (Figure 12.1). It can be argued that the role of the physiotherapist significantly overlaps with that of the occupational therapist and to a smaller extent that of the speech and language therapist. Many secondary care facilities treating PD in the UK have multidisciplinary teams, particularly departments of geriatric medicine. However, this is not universal and most neurologists struggle to refer their patients for such services as outpatients. In one survey of 72 consecutive PD patients attending a neurology clinic in 1995, only 29% had seen a physiotherapist, 18% an occupational therapist, and 15% a speech and language therapist. This low referral rate reflects multiple issues, including:

- the paucity of such therapy services in the UK which are already overburdened
- a perceived lack of data on the efficacy and effectiveness of paramedical therapies in PD.

These two major issues are linked – without adequate information on the value of paramedical therapies in PD, healthcare

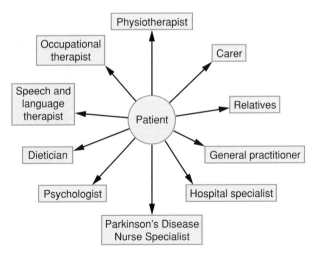

Figure 12.1
The multidisciplinary team in PD

purchasers will not invest in such services. It was with these considerations in mind that the Cochrane Movement Disorders Group was particularly keen to perform systematic reviews of the work of the main paramedical therapies, to document definitively what we know of their effects in PD and thus to inform better trial development in the future. This necessitated the rather artificial division of the individual therapies rather than examining the effects of multidisciplinary intervention, but was the only practical way to perform the reviews.

Physiotherapy

The purpose of physiotherapy in PD is to maximize functional ability and minimize secondary complications through movement rehabilitation within a context of education and support for the whole person (Plant *et al*). Many physiotherapy methods have been advocated in PD, including:

- proprioceptive neuromuscular facilitation – active muscle contractions, muscle stretch, patterns of movement, resistance, and verbal and visual cues mainly aimed at reducing rigidity
- Bobath – reducing abnormal muscle tone and posture using inhibiting techniques and postures, and facilitation of correct movement through handling by the therapist
- conductive education – reduction of dependency on aids and facilitation of participation in society
- ad hoc combinations of the above and other techniques
- miscellaneous methods such as karate, spinal flexibility exercises and balance training.

The Cochrane systematic review of any physiotherapy technique versus a placebo or sham intervention (often no intervention) located only 11 trials with 280 patients. Eight trials did not have adequate placebo treatments, all used a small number of patients, and the method of randomization and

concealment of allocation was good in only four trials. These methodological problems could potentially lead to bias from a number of sources. Although 10 trials claimed a positive effect from physiotherapy, few outcomes measured were statistically significant. Walking velocity was measured in four studies and increased significantly in two. However, there was significant heterogeneity in both trial design and the results due to the large positive effect of one inpatient trial, the remaining physiotherapy regimens being carried out in outpatient departments or at home. Stride length was the only other outcome measured in more than one trial; it significantly improved by 22% (two trials). Five other outcomes improved significantly in individual studies, but eight other outcomes did not.

The authors of the review concluded that, in view of the relatively small number of patients examined, the methodological flaws in most of the studies and the high likelihood of publication bias (as negative trials tend not to get published), there was insufficient evidence to support or refute the efficacy of physiotherapy in PD. They suggested that large well-designed placebo-controlled randomized control trials are needed to demonstrate the efficacy and effectiveness of physiotherapy in PD, with particular emphasis on the use of outcome measures with relevance to patients, carers, physicians and physiotherapists, and monitoring these for at least six months to determine the duration of any carryover effect.

The same group has performed the Cochrane review of one type of physiotherapy versus another. This found seven trials in 142 patients but, since there is no established 'gold standard' form of therapy against which to compare a novel type, these studies examined many varied types of therapy which could not be quantitatively summated. The individual studies were too small to demonstrate the superiority of one form of therapy over another, particularly considering their methodological flaws and possibility of publication bias.

It must be emphasized that the absence of evidence for a positive effect of physiotherapy in PD does not imply the absence of an effect. It means that further well-designed trials are needed to prove its effect. A Delphi project has been completed in the UK to reach a consensus on which physiotherapy technique(s) should be considered as 'standard'. These will now be compared in a well-designed trial with a control intervention. It is difficult from the existing evidence to perform a sample size calculation to decide how many patients will be required in a placebo-controlled study to avoid a false negative conclusion, but it is likely that 300–500 patients/arm will be needed.

Occupational therapy

Occupational therapists are trained to support individuals with PD to maintain their usual level of self-care, work and leisure activity for as long as possible. Interventions may include support in reorganizing the daily routine, learning new skills for alternative or adaptive ways to carry out activities, or providing and advising on specialist equipment or resources. When it is no longer possible to maintain patients' activities, occupational therapists support individuals in changing and adapting their roles. The aims of intervention are to reduce stress, minimize disability and handicap, and improve quality of life, despite the natural increase in impairment. The Cochrane systematic review of occupational therapy in PD found that only two randomized controlled trials had evaluated this in 84 patients. Although both trials reported positive effects of occupational therapy, major methodological criticisms (ie small numbers, inadequate placebo interventions, methods of randomization and concealment of allocation) and the possibility of publication bias led the authors to conclude that there is insufficient evidence to support or refute the efficacy of occupational therapy in PD.

As with physiotherapy, a systematic approach to occupational therapy development in PD is needed. A Delphi project is underway to ask individual therapists across the UK how they treat patients and what techniques they feel work best. Then, armed with this consensus, one or more large well-designed trials should be mounted to evaluate 'standard' occupational therapy versus a control intervention. Only then can alternative methods of occupational therapy be compared with the standard form.

Speech and language therapy
Dysarthria

Dysarthria is a common manifestation of PD which increases in frequency and intensity with progression of the disease. The term 'dysarthria' is a collective name for a group of speech disorders resulting from disturbances in muscular control of the speech mechanism due to damage of the central nervous system. These problems with oral communication stem from paralysis, weakness or incoordination of the speech musculature.

Common characteristics of parkinsonian dysarthria are:

- monotomy of pitch and volume (dysprosody)
- reduced stress
- imprecise articulation
- variations in speed, resulting in both inappropriate silences and rushes of speech
- a breathy hoarseness to the speech (hypophonia), reflecting the difficulty the patient has in synchronizing talking and breathing.

Many of these features are attributed to hypokinesia (paucity of movement).

The neural mechanisms underlying dysarthria in PD are poorly understood. Laryngeal examination by stroboscopy has shown asymmetric abductor and adductor movements and incomplete vocal cord closure in Parkinsonian patients. Bowed vocal cords, which are firm rather than flaccid, have been observed during speech and may be related to the increased rigidity in the vocalis muscle and to breathy phonation. Dysynchronous vocal cord motion has also been observed and is related to hoarseness.

The speech and language therapist can treat dysarthria in PD with behavioural treatment techniques, such as drills and exercises, and with instrumental aids including prosthetic and augmentative devices.

The Cochrane reviews of speech and language therapists in PD found three randomized controlled trials comparing speech and language therapy with placebo for speech disorders in only 63 patients with PD. However, numerical data were only available from two trials in just 41 patients. Also, changes in outcomes were not compared between the intervention and placebo groups; the authors compared baseline and final outcomes for each arm separately. Thus, in two studies the loudness of patients' voices was increased by 7–18%, depending on the speaking task being performed. It is likely that this was a clinically significant improvement. Although the degree of improvement reduced after six months, it was still within a clinically useful range. Other measures of dysarthria (eg monotonicity, pitch) were measured in two trials and also improved, although the clinical significance of these improvements was less clear-cut. The small numbers of patients, the methodological flaws in the trials and the possibility of publication bias prevented a conclusion from being made on the efficacy of speech and language therapists in PD. Much larger trials are required once a 'standard' approach to therapy has been agreed within the profession.

The Cochrane review comparing various types of speech and language therapy in PD found two trials in 71 patients. The types of therapy were so heterogenous that the results could not undergo meta-analysis but there was no conclusive evidence that one form of therapy was better than another, bearing in mind the small numbers and methodological criticisms of the studies.

> Cochrane reviews show that there is insufficient evidence to prove the efficacy of physiotherapy, occupational therapy, and speech and language therapy in PD

Dysphagia

Dysphagia occurs frequently in PD, although patients themselves may be unaware of swallowing difficulties. Several abnormalities in the various phases of swallowing have been described and include abnormal bolus formation, transfer and oesophageal dysmotility. Swallowing speed and bolus volume are significantly lower in patients when compared to age-matched controls, and decline significantly when disease severity (measured by the Hoehn and Yahr score, page 24) increases. Dysphagia can lead to 'silent aspiration', and although some authors have suggested that this leads to an increased risk of pneumonia which is a significant cause of mortality in patients with PD, others have found no association with dysphagia and chest infections requiring antibiotics.

Although levodopa improves swallowing speed, pharmacotherapy has only a limited amount to offer patients with more severe deficits. It has, therefore, been suggested that speech and language therapy may improve the remaining swallowing difficulties experienced by patients with PD. Therapists provide careful assessment and diagnosis of swallowing problems. They advise on swallowing technique, provide exercises, may offer dietary alternatives, and advise on food consistency to reduce the risks of ill health and promote safety and comfort in swallowing.

> Speech and language therapy may improve the swallowing difficulties that are not alleviated by pharmacotherapy

The Cochrane review of speech and language therapist for dysphagia failed to find any trials examining this issue, although the North

American 'Swallowing Trial' is looking at the use of thickened fluids and chin down posture in dementia and PD.

> Further trials are needed to assess the effects of interventions such as physiotherapy, occupational therapy, and speech and language therapy, and when they should be used. In the meantime, it would seem prudent to refer patients with advanced disease for assessment and treatment by a multidisciplinary team

PD Nurse Specialists (PDNSs)

The concept of PDNSs has been developed in the UK by a collaboration between the PD Society and the pharmaceutical industry. The first five PDNSs were introduced in the early 1990s but their success led to many other posts developing throughout the country, usually based in secondary care with a clinician with a particular interest in PD. At present, there are about 100 nurses in the UK, although the PD Society aims to increase this to 240.

> Support from the UK PD Society and the pharmaceutical industry has allowed the National Health Service (NHS) to expand to about 100 nurses nationwide, but a total of 240 will ultimately be needed to cover the whole country

PDNSs play a number of valuable roles:

- as a key worker, they provide a link between the patient and his or her carer with primary and secondary care clinicians and nurses, with paramedical therapists, and with social services.
- they are often in the best position to coordinate all aspects of the patient's 'care package'.
- they are trained to be able to advise patients on their medication within the limits set by medical staff, including more complex treatment regimens such as apomorphine injections and infusions.

- they can inform and educate patients, carers, other nurses and therapists, and medical staff about the condition and its treatment.

> PDNSs act as key workers to coordinate the patient's care package, advise on medication issues, and educate patients, carers, medical staff, and other nurses and therapists

There has been considerable debate about whether PDNSs should be based in the community or in secondary care. The precise location of their office or base probably does not matter provided their post allows them considerable access to patients in the community and access to expertise in the management of PD which is usually based in secondary care.

> PDNSs are best based in the community with strong links with specialist PD clinics in secondary care

The cost-effectiveness of the PDNSs has recently been evaluated in a randomized controlled trial in the UK. In nine randomly selected health authorities, stratified by population mortality rates and social deprivation, 438 general practitioners (GPs) recruited 1,859 patients with PD. Of these, 1,041 patients were allocated to receive the services of a PDSN (home visits at eight-week intervals), while 818 received standard care (control group). They were followed for two years using blinded raters who interviewed patients in their homes to record data on quality of life and health economics.

The original presentation of the results suggested that in the nurse group there was a statistically significant reduction in the number of fractures, improvement in quality of life, a reduced hospital admission rate, and a reduced length of institutional care. Although there were increased costs incurred by the nurse's salary and running costs, increased provision of benefits, increased drug costs and increased paramedical therapy provision, there was reduced expenditure on respite care, hospitalization and institutional care. The provision of a nurse saved £300/patient/year during the first year of the project. With a conservative case load of 150 parkinsonian patients, a nurse could save society about £45,000/annum. Due to the design of this study, these results can be generalized to the rest of the UK.

> PDNSs have been shown to be cost-effective and to improve quality of life in a large randomized controlled trial

However, the recent presentation of the final two-year results is at odds with the above. It failed to demonstrate any benefit from nurse input in mild or severe disease, but showed significantly reduced institutional care and mortality in moderate disease and a trend towards a reduction in costs. This is perhaps to be expected since mild patients will require little input from anyone and those with severe disease may well be institutionalized with few therapeutic options at that stage of the disease. In contrast, those with moderate disease have more complex problems which are amenable to intervention if the nurse encourages referrals for such treatment. Clarification of the results of this project are awaited when the full paper is published in the near future.

Other therapies

Other therapists may be required by patients with PD at various stages. The advice of a nutritionalist (dietitian), for example, can be invaluable as unexplained weight loss and dysphagia are common in the condition. Similarly, a continence nurse may be needed for bladder disturbance in patients with advanced disease. Furthermore, a psychologist may be required to advise patients on the management of anxiety which can be a problem at any stage of the condition.

Further reading

Clarke CE, Gullaksen E, MacDonald S, Lowe F. Referral criteria for speech and language therapy assessment of dysphagia caused by idiopathic Parkinsons disease. *Acta Neurol Scand* 1998; **97**: 27–35.

Clarke CE, Zobiw R, Gullaksen E. Quality of life and care in Parkinson's disease. *Br J Clin Pract* 1995; **49**: 288–93.

Deane KHO, Whurr R, Playford ED *et al*. Speech and language therapy for dysarthia in Parkinson's disease (Cochrane Reviews). In: *The Cochrane Library*; Issue 2. Oxford: Update Software, 2000.

Deane KHO, Ellis-Hill C, Clarke CE *et al*. Occupational therapy for patients with Parkinson's disease (Cochrane Revew). In: *The Cochrane Library*; Issue 3. Oxford: Update Software, 2001.

Deane KHO, Jones D, Clarke CE *et al*. Physiotherapy for patients with Parkinson's disease (Cochrane Revew). In: *The Cochrane Library*; Issue 3. Oxford: Update Software, 2001.

Findley L, Peto V, Pugner K *et al*. The impact of Parkinson's disease on quality of life: results of a research survey in the UK. *Mov Disord* 2000; **15**(suppl 3): 179.

Jarman B, Hurwitz B, Cook A. Parkinson's Disease Nurse Specialists in primary care: a randomised controlled trial. *Mov Disord* 2000; **15**(suppl 3): 178.

MacMahon DG, Findley L, Holmes J, Pugner K. The true economic impact of Parkinson's disease: a research survey in the UK. *Mov Disord* 2000; **15**(suppl 3): 178–9.

Plant RP, Jones D, Ashburn A *et al*. Evaluation of physiotherapy in Parkinson's disease: project update. The science and practice of multidisciplinary care in Parkinson's disease and Parkinsonism. London: British Geriatric Society, 1999.

13. Management guidelines

Formal management guidelines
Specific management problems

Table 13.2
Strength of recommendation for clinical decision-making

Strength	Recommendation
A	Directly based on category I evidence
B	Directly based on category II evidence or extrapolated recommendation from category I evidence
C	Directly based on category III evidence or extrapolated recommendation from category I or II evidence
D	Directly based on category IV evidence or extrapolated recommendation from category I, II or III evidence

Formal management guidelines

A number of management guidelines for idiopathic Parkinson's Disease (PD) have been published over the past decade, stimulated particularly by the drive towards clinical decisions becoming evidence-based. However, the two treatment algorithms devised by the American Academy of Neurology and the primary and secondary care guidelines devised in the UK were prepared following consensus conferences without systematic review of the literature and with no weighting of the evidence in terms of quality (Tables 13.1 and 13.2). These latter elements are crucial to the development of reliable guidelines as exemplified by the Scottish Intercollegiate

Guideline Network's (SIGN) guidelines on the management of epilepsy and other conditions. It is accepted that in too many areas no evidence exists for recommendations to be made and in such situations the clinical experience of an expert panel is all that can be provided. However, this process must be explicit in any series of guidelines.

Specific management problems

Figure 13.1 outlines the latest guidelines for the management of PD, which are also mentioned below. This is influenced by my own opinions in places and where this is the case is stated clearly and the alternatives discussed.

Diagnosis

All patients with suspected PD should be referred to a neurologist or a geriatrician with experience in diagnosing the disease before they are treated – this will improve the diagnostic accuracy rate and ensure the latest views on treatment and support are provided to the patient. The latter may involve counselling by a Parkinson's Disease Nurse Specialist (page 89). While these recommendations are generally accepted, there is no trial work to support them other than that on misdiagnosis performed by several PD brain banks. The problem of long waiting lists for specialist referral in the UK can be surmounted by referring the patient to a specialist movement

Table 13.1
Categories of evidence for clinical decision-making

Category	Type of evidence
Ia	Evidence from systematic reviews of randomized controlled trials
Ib	Evidence from one or more randomized controlled trials
IIa	Evidence from one or more controlled but non-randomized study
IIb	Evidence from one or more quasi-experimental study
III	Evidence from descriptive study(s) such as case-control
IV	Evidence from expert committee reports or opinions or clinical experience of respected authorities

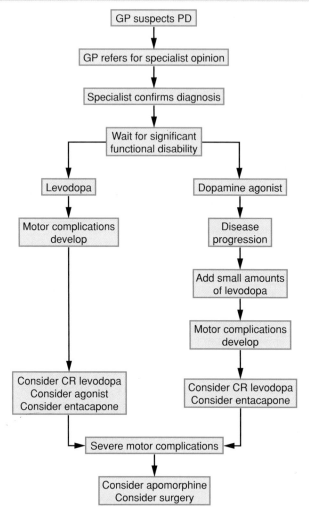

Figure 13.1
Guidelines for the management of PD. Adapted from Bhatia *et al. Hosp Med* 1998; **59**: 469-80

disorders clinic which may have a shorter waiting time.

Early disease

In the absence of further quality of life and health economics data, it is unclear whether or not the ability of dopamine agonists to delay motor complications in early disease compared with levodopa is worthwhile. A pragmatic policy must therefore be adopted. In very young (20–40 years) patients, a policy of agonist

monotherapy can be supported. On the other hand, in those with significant co-morbidity, a short life expectancy or complex polypharmacy, a case can be made for using levodopa. Most patients lie between these extremes. Unless the patient will consider joining studies such as the PD MED trial, decisions for this group must rest on a frank discussion between the patient, the carer and the clinician, bearing in mind factors such as the need to work which may be better fostered in the short-term by using levodopa.

Once the decision has been made to introduce levodopa, the dose should be restricted to the lowest needed to maintain the patient's quality of life. Initially, this may only require 100 mg levodopa (with an aromatic amino acid decarboxylase inhibitor) tid with main meals – elderly patients may even require only one-half of this dose. The dose can be increased conveniently by adding 100 mg doses at mid-morning coffee and then mid-afternoon tea. This fractionation may reduce the propensity to develop motor complications, but no hard evidence for this exists. Evidence from two trials demonstrates that there is no point in using the more expensive controlled-release formulations at this stage as they generate complications at the same rate as immediate-release levodopa preparations.

> Once the decision has been made to introduce levodopa, the dose should be restricted to the lowest required to maintain the patient's quality of life

The adverse event profiles of the anticholinergics and amantadine are such that they should not be used as monotherapy. Anticholinergics may be used for severe tremor but even then many will develop confusion. Amantadine can be used for dyskinesia (discussed below).

The role of selegiline as monotherapy is unclear and further work is needed regarding its efficacy on motor impairments and whether it increases or decreases mortality. This drug is included in the PD MED trial.

Motor complications

Many patients on levodopa monotherapy are still referred to clinics, having developed motor complications (Figure 13.2). The first approach should be to fractionate the dose of levodopa and lower each dose. For example, Sinemet 275 tid becomes Sinemet Plus taken six times daily. Care should be taken not to reduce the dose too much at each time interval as this may not

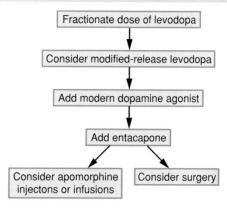

Figure 13.2
Managing motor complications

reach the therapeutic threshold. An alternative is to replace or add modified-release levodopa to the standard preparation. Suggestions for conversion are given in chapter 7.

The benefit obtained from adding a dopamine agonist at this stage seems greater than that from adding entacapone, although direct comparitor studies have not been performed. It would, therefore, seem prudent to add a modern agonist (ie cabergoline, pergolide, pramipexole, ropinirole) first and then entacapone when further deterioration and complications develop. This leads to a 'triple therapy' approach.

If the patient continues to suffer from severe and frequent 'off' periods despite the above changes then initially intermittent apomorphine injections may be appropriate, leading to continuous apomorphine infusion if necessary. This will require referral to a centre able to provide and monitor an apomorphine service.

Occasionally, severe 'off' periods will respond to moving all protein to the evening meal. This reduces the competition for absorption between dietary amino acids and levodopa during the day but will make the evenings worse. For patients with severe dyskinesia, continuous apomorphine infusion is an alternative to surgical intervention.

Surgery

In the absence of adequate data from randomized controlled trials, it is impossible to be dogmatic about which surgical procedure should be offered to which patient. However, guidelines have been drawn up by a task force on surgery for PD established by the American Academy of Neurology (Table 13.3).

It is clear that thalamotomy and thalamic stimulation only affect tremor, so these techniques should be restricted to PD patients with severe rest tremor, and little else, which is unresponsive to changes in pharmacotherapy. No information on the relative merits of thalamic lesion versus stimulation is available in terms of quality of life or cost-benefit.

Concern that lesioning procedures are irreversible compared to stimulation has led many to abandon further work with pallidotomy and more recently subthalamotomy. The additional benefit with STN stimulation of a large reduction in medication has the added bonuses of potentially reduced dyskinesia in the long-term and reduced drug costs. Stimulation can also be performed safely in both hemispheres, unlike pallidotomy. Against this is the additional cost of stimulation and the frequent need to re-programme the pulse generator. Without further data on the effects of these procedures on quality of life and health economics, it is impossible to provide any firm guidance on patient or procedure selection.

Intracerebral grafting in PD (chapter 11) remains experimental and should be restricted to a small number of experienced units.

Paramedical therapies and nursing care

There is insufficient trial evidence on the effects in PD of physiotherapy, occupational therapy, speech and language therapy for dysarthria and dysphagia to reach any firm conclusions about whether or not and when they should be used. However, most clinicians would consider referring patients with more advanced disease for a multidisciplinary assessment and possible treatment by such therapists. There is early evidence that patients with moderately severe PD benefit from the input of a PD Nurse Specialist.

Non-motor complications

The management of individual non-motor problems such as depression, dementia and psychosis is discussed in chapter 10.

Further reading

Bhatia K, Brooks D, Burn D et al. Guidelines for the management of Parkinson's disease. *Hosp Med* 1998; **59**: 469–80.

Table 13.3
American Academy of Neurology guidelines for surgery in PD

Procedure	Bradykinesia	Tremor	Dyskinesia	Recommendation	Strength of recommendation*
Unilateral thalamotomy	No	Yes	No	Safe, effective	C
Bilateral thalamotomy	No	Yes	No	Doubtful	D
Unilateral pallidotomy	Yes	Yes	Yes	Safe, effective	C
Bilateral pallidotomy	Yes	Yes	Yes	Doubtful	D
Unilateral thalamic stimulation	No	Yes	No	Safe, effective	C
Bilateral thalamic stimulation	No	Yes	No	Investigational	
Bilateral pallidal stimulation	Yes	Yes	Yes	Investigational	
Bilateral STN stimulation	Yes	Yes	Yes	Investigational	
Fetal implant	Yes	Yes	Yes	Investigational	

*(see Table 13.2)

Hallett M, Litvan I, The Task Force on Surgery for Parkinson's Disease. Evaluation of surgery for Parkinson's disease. *Neurology* 1999; **53**: 1910–21.

Koller WC, Silver DE, Lieberman A. An algorithm for the management of Parkinson's disease. *Neurology* 1994; **44**(suppl 10): S1-52.

MacMahon DG, Thomas S. Practical approach to quality of life in Parkinson's disease. *J Neurol* 1998; **245**: S19-22.

Olanow CW, Koller WC. An algorithm (decision tree) for the managment of Parkinson's disease. *Neurology* 1998; **50**(suppl 3): S1-57.

Scottish Intercollegiate Guideline Network (SIGN) website: http://www.sign.ac.uk.

Shekelle PG, Woolf SH, Eccles M, Grimshaw J. Developing guidelines. *BMJ* 1999; **318**: 593–6.

Useful addresses and information

Charities
Reference books
Websites

Charities

Parkinson's Disease Society of the United
Kingdom
215 Vauxhall Bridge Road
London SW1V 1EJ
Tel: (0)20 7931 8080
Fax: (0)20 7233 9908
E-mail: mailbox@pdsuk.demon.co.uk
Helpline: 0808 800 0303

Parkinson's Disease Society Scotland
Scottish Resource
10 Claremont Terrace
Glasgow G3 7XR
Tel/Fax: (0)141 332 3343

Parkinson's Association of Ireland
Carmichael House
North Brunswick Street
Dublin 7
Tel: 03531 8722234
Fax: 03531 8735737

YAPPRS (Young Active Parkinsonians, Partners
and Relatives)
c/o Emma Bennion
Church Farm
Bircham Newton
King's Lynn
Norfolk PE31 6QZ
Tel/Fax: (0)1485 578592

European Parkinson's Disease Association
EPDA Liaison
c/o Lizzie Graham
215 Vauxhall Bridge Road
London SW1V 1EJ
Tel: (0)20 7932 1304
Fax: (0)20 7233 9226
E-mail: lizzie@epda.demon.co.uk

Reference books

Quinn NP, ed. *Parkinsonism*. London: Bailliere
    Tindall, 1997.
Watts RL, Koller WC, eds. *Movement disorders:
    neurologic principles and practice*. New York:
    McGraw-Hill, 1997.

Websites

Awakenings site of European Parkinson's
Disease Association – useful for staff and
patients: http://www.parkinsonsdisease.com.

Cochrane Collaboration:
http://www.cochrane.org

Information service for patients:
http://www.parkinsonsinfo.com

Information service for younger patients:
http://www.young-parkinsons.org.uk.

Teaching material for paramedical staff:
http://www.dna2z.com

Index

Page numbers in *italics* refer to information that is shown only in a table or figure